YOU, BUT BETTER

STOP MAKING YOUR HEALTH SO HARD!

KELLY MORGAN, PH.D.

Copyright © 2019; 2022 by Kelly Morgan, Ph.D.

All rights reserved.

No part of this book may be reproduced in any form or by any electronic or mechanical means, including information storage and retrieval systems, without written permission from the author, except for the use of brief quotations in a book review.

Cover designed by MiblArt

Health is the ability to have energy and vigor of body, mind, or spirit—not being feeble or sick.

Wellness is a balance of the mind, body, and spirit that leads to a general feeling of well-being.

INTRODUCTION

Have you ever just needed a break? Some time to get away from life, stress, and the pressures of always achieving? I did. And I did it in the most extreme way possible, because I'm just that kind of girl.

I won't bore you with the details of why my life got out of control, mostly because they just sound silly when I say them out loud. But that's the problem, because "silly" things add up. I kept adding one more thing to my schedule and list of what I need to do to be the ultimate version of myself. It felt so hard to keep it all together—especially being healthy and happy. I was gradually ruining my life, and I was taking those closest to me down the rabbit hole as well.

I'm genetically predisposed to panic attacks, but they only tend to rear their ugly heads about twice a year, and usually for a good reason. My panic attacks began to increase in frequency, but they were happening for no apparent reason. Except, anyone else could tell you that the reason was that I over-complicated everything and set unreasonable goals for myself.

I talked myself into thinking I was going crazy. I'm not one to do things halfway, you see. I decided that what I needed was a trip to outpatient therapy at a local mental hospital. Yes. For real.

When I imagined this, I saw a pool, spa food, and a lot of talking about my feelings. I thought I could get this nice break where I could feel refreshed. Basically, I pictured a fancy spa in Sedona.

It was nothing like that. I got myself the heck out before lunchtime, because I wasn't mentally ill—I was stressed, burned out, too hard on myself, and making life way too hard. I got to this point because I kept telling myself and everyone around me whose concern was growing that "I'm fine!" Honey, I wasn't fine. I wasn't "outpatient therapy not fine," but I was suffering from burnout that I tried to smooth over with Netflix marathons, pizza, and generally anti-social behavior because I just couldn't even. That all changed when I finally figured out how to approach my life, happiness, health, and overall wellness in a way that doesn't make it so hard. It's okay not to be fine. It's what you do about it that matters.

Is "I'm fine" *your* automatic answer to someone asking how you are, despite really feeling tired, overwhelmed, and so on?

You're totally normal. We women tend to brush aside our feelings, stress, and health concerns in favor of politeness and continually putting others before ourselves. We put our health aside not only to care for other people, but to start achieving other things in our lives. Maybe we want to go to grad school, to save up for a home, to move to a new city. Whatever it may be, I find that many women are so focused on all these other goals in their lives that they keep putting off their health.

Even when you're not focused on other people, there's also the task of simply keeping your life together. I'm talking about your work, social life, volunteering, all these other things that are important to you.

Let's begin with a simple question: When was the last time

you felt amazing? There's been a time in all of our lives where we've been really healthy. We've really been great, for real. We've all had that success before, so we know it's possible. Maybe you've been putting aside getting back to that feeling because you're in your 20s, 30s, or 40s, and you keep telling yourself, "Oh, I don't have any health concerns; I'm still young."

As you stop taking care of yourself to take care of everything else in life, you make it a little bit more difficult to get back to what you deserve—feeling great. You deserve that energy. You deserve to be feeling awesome.

Take stock of the last time you felt really good. Think about the last time you felt like you were in charge of your health, because that also means that you had everything going right, you felt well, you had the energy. Then think about what was going on. Usually it means that you were happy, you were well-rested, you were eating well, you were moving around. Taking stock of exactly what that feeling felt like and when you felt it, you can have that serve as the answer to "What are we working toward?"

How do we get back to feeling that way? The version of you when you last felt great is your goal. Now, take a look at your current lifestyle and find some places you can make little tweaks. Can you maybe add some vegetables to dinner or have one night where you don't get takeout? Remember to take baby steps. And then just keep adding on the good and/or removing the unhelpful, seeing what sticks until you begin feeling great again.

Pick one thing that could get you toward that feeling again. Set your alarm earlier or you could pack some carrot sticks, or you could take five minutes where everybody has to leave you alone. Whatever it is, take one baby step toward that feeling so you can match up your current reality with that healthier version of yourself.

Not only is your likelihood of success higher if you focus on just one thing, but because you're experimenting, you can see what works first and then add something else.

But, big sweeping changes don't work. I've done it; it doesn't work. I promise. You will fail, and I don't want you to fail—I want you to feel awesome.

You deserve to feel great! Your body is just dying to feel great. In fact, being healthy is not complicated—you don't have to be on a special diet, you don't have to do a certain workout routine. What you need to do is whatever it is that fits in your crazy life, because most of your life is not going to change. Your lifestyle is your lifestyle—whether it's force of habit, necessity, or you simply like it that way. Don't assume making changes to your health, whatever those may be, requires that you change the rest of your life, because you're not going to. It isn't realistic.

There's an easier way to make sustainable and manageable lifestyle changes, and I'm going to help you take that easier path to long-term success.

I'm Dr. Kelly Morgan, your health coach and personal champion. I help busy, high-achieving women gain control of their health and use it as a tool for continuing to lead their crazy lives and achieve their big dreams. I do this through teaching real-life, no-fluff ways to find a sustainable and manageable healthy lifestyle that works in your current life without making drastic changes. For real this time.

I've experienced both poor and fabulous health. I have recovered from anorexia, gained too much weight in a time of stress, and lost the weight to get to a happy place, finally. I know what it takes to find balance while fulfilling the seemingly endless work, academic, family, social, and personal commitments we all have.

You might have noticed that I'm a fellow overachiever. This is good news for you because I can use my experience as a certified health coach, personal trainer, group fitness instructor, nutrition fitness specialist, and yoga teacher as well as years as a health professor to help you. I have a near-100 percent success rate with helping my clients and students through this same program.

We're going to do this whole process together, step by step. I developed this program to address both your health and your wellness to help you feel your best and have healthy habits that fit into your already crazy life without major changes. Why? Because big, sweeping changes just plain don't work. This book will show you the exact system I have used with hundreds of clients and students. I know from their experiences that this proven program will give you the kick in the pants you need to start making changes that fit into your life.

The key factor in your success is you. Only you know what exactly you want to achieve and what you are (or aren't) willing to do to get there. The core of this book is to guide you into and through creating a program and lifestyle that is significant, important, and relevant to you (so you find reason to follow through) and matches how you want to live your life (so you'll keep doing it).

This book is designed to help you tailor your plan to your wants, needs, and lifestyle. I believe that you're only motivated to keep up with what works in the context of your life. So, these tools will guide you to design your unique plan of action, get your mindset right, figure out your food and exercise, and, most importantly, manage your stress and energy. Additionally, I've provided everything you need to get started on a no-nonsense exercise and meal plan that will work for you—without alienating you from your family and friends. We're talking no weird or intense diet and exercise plans. Only tools that work.

The strategies I'm giving you in this book are based on research and proven methodologies. We'll use real, honest-to-goodness methods and solutions to get you where you want to be in the most reasonable and efficient way. Real strategies that work, when combined with a program that best fits you and your life, lead to success.

This program includes sections devoted to my seven pillars of a healthy lifestyle and has all the information you need to set your personal goals, create a bullet-proof plan, learn only what is necessary (no fluff guarantee!), and take action immediately. Along with these pillars, there are worksheets that will help you delve deeper into your plan as well as keep you organized. You can see them right here in the book or download them in a the free program workbook from my website at www.tsirona.com/ybbbook or by scanning the QR code below:

I have also written a companion journal and workbook that will help you gain the insight to develop a sustainable and manageable healthy lifestyle strategy to fit your individual needs. The journal prompts and exercises help you expand on this approach. If you're interested, scan the QR code below or go to: https://amzn.to/3Q7iBYG

Introduction

What's in This Book?

I like to know what I'm doing before I start. That's why I'd like to give you the game plan for the rest of this book (and for your healthy lifestyle success story).

We'll start with my first pillar of health, **Self-Examination**. In this pillar, we'll get to the real star of this story—you. Essentially, we'll go spelunking into your beliefs, attitudes, and behaviors and what they all mean for your goals. When we come out the other end, we'll have a better idea of what you want to achieve in your plan and, most importantly, why. We will then discuss how to set your goals and determine your milestones along the way in the second pillar, Goal Setting.

Along with Self-Examination, **Goal Setting** is a key pillar that will be the difference between what hasn't stuck in the past and getting to the new you. It involves the majority of the prework needed for you to have a healthier future lifestyle that you won't have to think about. After completing these pillars, you'll have the all-important awareness needed to recognize exactly what you want to change and what you need to do so. We'll transform the areas you think need attention into Specific, Measurable, Attainable, Relevant, and Time-bound (SMART) goals. Included in this pillar are the nitty-gritty details on tracking your progress and measuring your goals over time so you can see your changes in real-time.

The third pillar we'll tackle is your **Mindset**. This pillar fortifies you to take on the serious goals and plans you came up with in your goal setting. If it were easy to do all of this, you probably would have done it before. In this pillar, we're going to get your mind in the right place by focusing on useful outlooks that meld your high-achieving superpowers with tools for keeping perfectionism and negativity in check.

Before moving on to the rest of the program, we'll take a brief pit stop in the **A Moment on Weight Loss** section. Though this isn't a weight loss book, many readers will likely have weight loss as one of their goals. We'll dispel misinformation and rumors, and you'll get the real information on weight loss that you can use if it happens to be one of your goals.

By the time we get to the **Movement** pillar, we're really trucking. I'll help you choose a manageable activity routine that gets you moving more while fitting into your unique lifestyle, no matter your preferences, needs, or barriers. If you're interested in setting fitness goals, I will break down exercises so you feel knowledgeable and comfortable with each activity. We'll get you set up with exercises that can be done with whatever equipment, time, resources, or limitations you may have. Exercise can be anything you want it to be, as long as you're moving.

While exercising is crucial, you can't talk about movement without **Nutrition**. This pillar covers basic nutrition for real people and guidelines to follow whether you're a sedentary desk worker or an elite athlete. We'll also get into mindful eating and how to prevent emotional eating triggers from derailing your progress. I've included meal plans that you can use as-written or tweak to fit your preferences.

Like movement and nutrition, the next two pillars go hand-in-hand. The **Stress Management** pillar is all about understanding what causes stress and how to use that knowledge to help you manage it. We'll also talk about some techniques you can use to stop stressful, destructive thought patterns from making your life harder. We'll close out this pillar with ideas for self-care, relaxation, and finding people who can love on you and make everything easier.

Stress is one of the biggest problems when it comes to managing energy, so the **Energy Management** pillar is a close relative of stress management. In this pillar, we'll talk about your energy cycle and limitations. Because your energy is finite, we'll also discuss not forcing yourself to "do it all," no matter how much of the world is on your shoulders. We'll discuss quality sleep as a key way to replenish energy as well as some tricks to keep your energy up throughout the day.

Finally, you'll reach the **Now What?** section that is all about what happens after you have reached and exceeded your goals and are beginning to set new ones. Your health and wellness are constantly evolving because of your interests, lifestyle, changing goals, and age. This section will give you everything you need to stay agile and adapt to life beyond your initial goals.

How to Use This Book

You can use this book in any manner that you find useful. The pillars in the program can take as long as you need or be repeated. There are no rules here. Furthermore, you can read each pillar as you go, working on each in real-time. You can also read everything all at once and go back to each pillar as you're ready.

Do what you need, how you need. Now, let's get crackin' on making big changes to your health!

Recommended Schedule

I recommend that you plan completion dates for each part of the program to keep yourself accountable. These dates can be changed as needed, but defining a schedule will help you plan the time needed for each pillar and keep you on track.

To hold yourself accountable, list the date by which you will complete each portion. Remember, be reasonable with yourself. It's not a sprint. You can download a free workbook with a schedule worksheet at www.tsirona.com/ybbbook or by scanning the QR code below:

Let's get started, shall we?

PILLAR ONE: SELF-ORIENTATION

Getting to Know Yourself

This program is all about you. We start with this first pillar, Self-Orientation, because you need to know yourself really well to create the perfect plan. This pillar will be an interesting one, because it requires introspection into who you are at a deep level. To create lasting change in this program, you need to stay true to who you are.

Your World View

Your worldview is made up of your experiences, education, upbringing, attitudes, values, and beliefs. Though many of us share parts of our worldviews and can find common ground, everyone's perception of how the world works and her place in it is unique. Perception is everything, and we're going to start our goal-setting work by understanding what you perceive to be true.

Values and beliefs are part of our core selves, and they are not easily changed. They come from a lifetime of experience, communication with people in our lives, and education. Your values are ideas that reflect what you deem most important in life—equality and loyalty, for example. They can be consciously chosen through your experiences and they can also be lived out unconsciously, like those values you learned at such an early age from your family that you don't remember having learned them.

When you identify and acknowledge your values, you can set goals that honor them. By understanding the underlying priorities in your life, you'll be able to determine the best direction for you and your goals and, essentially, stand "on-brand" with yourself. When we live according to our values, we feel consistent and fulfilled.

To help identify your values, I've provided a few questions to get you thinking. Be honest, and think about what is deeply important to you. This worksheet is also in the free program workbook on my website at www.tsirona.com/ybbbook (see the QR code in the Introduction).

What is most important to you in life? Make a list of at least five things you feel passionately about. This does not have to be about your health. Think big picture.

Here is a list of common core values from Carnegie Mellon University. Circle or mark the ones that resonate with you.

You, but Better

Abundance	Daring	Intuition	Preparedness
Acceptance	Decisiveness	Joy	Proactivity
Accountability	Dedication	Kindness	Professionalism
Achievement	Dependability	Knowledge	Punctuality
Advancement	Diversity	Leadership	Recognition
Adventure	Empathy	Learning	Relationships
Advocacy	Encouragement	Love	Reliability
Ambition	Enthusiasm	Loyalty	Resilience
Appreciation	Ethics	Mindfulness	Resourcefulness
Attractiveness	Excellence	Motivation	Responsibility
Autonomy	Expressiveness	Optimism	Responsiveness
Balance	Fairness	Open-Mindedness	Security
Being the Best	Family	Originality	Self-Control
Benevolence	Friendships	Passion	Selflessness
Boldness	Flexibility	Performance	Simplicity
Brilliance	Freedom	Personal Development	Stability
Calmness	Fun		Success
Caring	Generosity	Proactive	Teamwork
Challenge	Grace	Professionalism	Thankfulness
Charity	Growth	Quality	Thoughtfulness
Cheerfulness	Flexibility	Recognition	Traditionalism
Cleverness	Happiness	Risk Taking	Trustworthiness
Community	Health	Safety	Understanding
Commitment	Honesty	Security	Uniqueness
Compassion	Humility	Service	Usefulness
Cooperation	Humor	Spirituality	Versatility
Collaboration	Inclusiveness	Stability	Vision
Consistency	Independence	Peace	Warmth
Contribution	Individuality	Perfection	Wealth
Creativity	Innovation	Playfulness	Well-Being
Credibility	Inspiration	Popularity	Wisdom
Curiosity	Intelligence	Power	Zeal

Of the values you marked, which are the three most important to you? When determining a path to success, keep these top three values in mind. For example, if you chose community, accountability, and relationships, you may find motivation by joining an exercise group or online support group. If you chose values like achievement and success, you may want to be extra vigilant with tracking your progress so you can see small successes as they happen. Your primary values will indicate the best way for you to approach this program.

While your values help guide your behavior, your beliefs are the assumptions you make about the world. They come from your experiences, and your belief system can grow as you mature through new experiences. These beliefs help to construct your view of yourself and your world, and we will use these beliefs as the scaffolding for your plan.

To get an idea of your beliefs, I've provided a few questions to get you thinking. Be honest when answering the questions below. Do not self-censor. Write what you truly believe. This worksheet is also in the free program workbook on my website at www.tsirona.com/ybbbook (see the QR code in the Introduction).

1. My definition of "health" is:
2. When if comes to my health, I am:
3. My future is:
4. My definition of "wellness" is:
5. Unhealthy people are:
6. Healthy people are:
7. I am not where I want to be with my health because:
8. True or false and why: My health is in my control.
9. True or false and why: I can make health behavior changes.
10. True or false and why: Being low-energy and unhealthy is a common problem.
11. True or false and why: I am at risk for health complications because of my lifestyle.
12. True or false and why: Maintaining a healthy lifestyle is the responsibility of the individual.

What did you notice in your responses? Is your outlook positive? Are you in control of your health? If you were to step outside of yourself to evaluate your beliefs, are any of these faulty? For example, are any based on body dysmorphia, fear, or something else that may not be grounded in reality? If you find any of your beliefs to be faulty or unhelpful, you may want to talk them through with a trusted friend. You can only be successful with change when you're true to who you are and your plan is based on the beliefs that will help you succeed.

Your character and actions are a result of your beliefs and values. Examine those beliefs and values closely in order to know yourself. This worksheet is also in the free program workbook on my website at www.tsirona.com/ybbbook (see the QR code in the Introduction).

Answer the questions below as honestly as possible:

1. What or who is the origin of my beliefs and values?
2. What are they based on? Am I using reliable evidence?
3. Do my actions reflect these beliefs and values?
4. Do my beliefs align with my values?
5. How have my beliefs and values evolved over the years?
6. How do they help me live a contented, happy life?

The other part of your worldview that is important in creating the new you is your attitudes. Attitudes come from your beliefs, and they are the mental tendencies you have toward yourself, others, circumstances, and the world. They are important because they help determine your decisions and behaviors alongside your values and beliefs.

The questions below will give you an idea of your attitudes about your health. These will help you when you choose goals and formulate your plan. Staying true to yourself makes for a successful plan. This worksheet is also in the free program workbook on my website at www.tsirona.com/ybbbook (see the QR code in the Introduction).

1. What words would you use to describe a "healthy" person? How do they look? How do they feel? What is their daily life like?

2. How do you feel physically? Consider how you feel now and how you have felt recently.
3. When did you last feel great physically? What changed?
4. How would you like to feel physically?
5. How do you feel mentally/emotionally?
6. How would you like to feel mentally/emotionally?
7. When did you last feel great mentally/emotionally? What changed?
8. What do you want to be able to do that you don't feel like you can do with your current body health state, or lifestyle?
9. What behaviors or situations got you to this point? In other words, what led you to pick up this book?
10. How can you change, replace, or eliminate those behaviors or situations? Write freely. These don't have to be strategies you'll implement now or ever.
11. What changes are you willing to make? What are you not willing to change/what can't you change?
12. Within what time period do you need to see changes in order to stay motivated?
13. Considering those changes, your timetable, and your lifestyle, list some strategies for making those changes.

Now, highlight words in your responses that stick out to you. Maybe you're using the same words and phrases over and over. Maybe you see something in there that you would like to incorporate into your goals. What is different between your answers about your current physical and mental or emotional state and where you would like to be? Note these things, but don't judge yourself.

Your Beliefs in Practice

Would you ever have the nerve to tell someone they look fat today? Of course not! What about getting on your best friend about eating a muffin instead of a high-protein breakfast? Doubtful. If it would be impolite, mean, or sometimes just plain ludicrous to put people down about their health and behaviors, why would you say such things to yourself?

I have a family member who jokingly refers to himself as "a big tub of goo." Sure, that's a funny mental picture, but the more he says those types of things to himself or others, the more he and everyone else will believe it. There's a concept of talking something into reality. The more time and power you give words, the more likely that belief or perception is to become reality. Think of urban legends that get told over and over until everyone starts to believe them.

Bottom line: you can talk both good and bad beliefs into reality. We are everything we think we are. It's not magic—it's just how our minds work. If you want to make changes in your life, you have to change both your thoughts and habits to be successful. Now, you don't need to lie to yourself and tell yourself over and over that you're a perfect goddess if you don't really believe it. But, anything you do say about yourself needs to be put in a positive light. It's useful to tell yourself that you have every tool you need to get to where you need to be with your goals. However, it's completely counterproductive to tell yourself continually that you have had every opportunity to get to your goal, but that you're too lazy, weak, or whatever to accomplish it. Don't let your own rhetoric defeat you. What a shame that would be!

We're going to work on this skill of talking the best of your beliefs into reality by identifying everything you like about yourself. If that's hard for you, think about the compliments others have given you. Put aside any negative self-talk or insecurities and brag about yourself for a moment.

For this exercise, you'll need to put pen to paper or fingers to keys. Just let it flow. Don't self-edit or review as you write. You're awesome, right? This doesn't change depending on how much yoga you do or how much lean muscle mass you have. Find a safe place to tuck this list away. You'll want to add to it as you progress through this program and discover more of your wonderful qualities. This worksheet is also in the free program workbook on my website at www.tsirona.com/ybbbook (see the QR code in the Introduction).

This time, you're going to list everything you want for yourself. Everything. Again, don't reread, edit, or censor what you write. There will be time for editing and analysis later. This process may take a few minutes or a few days. Either way, be sure you write down everything you hope for, no matter how outrageous. This worksheet is also in the free program workbook on my website at www.tsirona.com/ybbbook (see the QR code in the Introduction).

Stages of Change

Before you start setting goals and planning, you need to know how ready you are to make changes. Sure, your doctor may have told you that you need to find ways to reduce your stress or lower your blood pressure. Maybe you're even thinking it's the "right thing to do." Unless you're actually ready—wholeheartedly set—to make a big health change, you will not be compelled to stick with a plan and reach the goals you've decided on. And that's true no matter how good your plan is and how much you push yourself.

Everyone goes through five stages of change when they want to achieve a goal, which we will discuss in just a moment. In this section, we will figure out your stage of change so you know your starting point. If you haven't done anything to work toward a healthy lifestyle before and you're just now considering it, your goals and plan will be different from someone who has already been looking into ways to make healthy changes or from the person who has started down the path. We each have our own starting point, or stage of change.

The five stages of change are pre-contemplation, contemplation, preparation, action, and maintenance. Take a look at the statements below and figure out which stage of change you fall into for the changes you'd like to make in this program.

Pre-Contemplation (This is most likely not where you are since you're reading this, but it can be helpful to see what it would look like if you were not at all ready to do this.)

- I do not see my health behavior as a problem.
- I am not interested in discussing this with others that do see the behavior as a problem, like my doctor, friends, family members, or loved ones.
- I have no intention of changing my health behavior.
- I am unaware of the risks associated with not making a change or can easily rationalize them away.
- I have made previous attempts to change, feel hopeless about changing my health, and am not interested in trying again.

Contemplation

- I am aware of the need to change my health behavior.
- I am beginning to realize the risks of my health behavior.
- I am actively weighing the pros and cons of my health behavior.

- I am aware of the need for change, but I sometimes waver in my willingness to change.

Preparation

- I believe that my health behavior can be changed and that I can manage the change.
- I have made some successful attempts to change in the past.
- I intend to change.
- I clearly see the benefits of changing my health behavior.

Action

- I have already begun to make the behavior change.
- I am emotionally, intellectually, and behaviorally prepared to make the change consistently.
- I have a commitment to change.
- I have developed plans to maintain change.

Maintenance (This is your ending point, the goal, the holy grail!)

- My new health behaviors have been practiced consistently for over six months.
- My new behavior is becoming habitual.
- I have confidence in my ability to continue to change.

Changing is hard. There's no way around that. If it were easy, we'd all be healthy, happy, and dancing with unicorns. In fact, research shows that only about 20 percent of people with a less-than-ideal behavior are prepared to take action on making a change at any one time (9). Now that you've determined what stage you are in, here is your starting point:

- **Pre-Contemplation:** You may have picked this book up at the urging of someone else. Or, maybe you just wanted to read it for fun. If you are in the pre-contemplation stage, this is a good time for you to absorb the information in this book and decide if any change to your health or if any part of this program is your cup of tea. You would benefit from reading this book in its entirety or skipping around to sections that catch your eye. Your choice. You do you, my friend.
- **Contemplation:** You're at a crucial point in this stage. You will benefit from taking the assessments in the following chapters and doing a little free writing about what you want to feel like, health-wise, in the near- and long-term. You may feel a little indecisive right now, and that's fine! Change is difficult and can be life-altering, so you will want to nail down what you are considering changing and exactly why it would benefit you to do so. You may even want to just take some small steps toward changing the everyday activities you do: walk a little farther from the parking lot to the store, add in a serving of vegetables—easy stuff. These small changes will add up and give you a taste of what making a change would be like for you. You would benefit from reading the book in its entirety and taking notes of what catches your eye along the way. When you're ready, go back and take the book pillar-by-pillar, implementing each completely before moving to the next one.

- **Preparation:** If you are in the preparation stage, you're already convinced that you can start and finish a plan that would lead you to better health that fits into your life. For you, it will mostly be about continuing to be motivated and challenged in your new lifestyle. You know you can do it, so you'll mostly be challenged to *want* to continue doing it. The biggest step for you will be finding a way to make lifestyle changes that fit with what you are not only willing to do, but are comfortable enough doing so that your plan becomes your new lifestyle. You would benefit from taking this book one pillar at a time and implementing each stage fully before moving to the next one.
- **Action:** Well, look at you! You're already in motion, so this plan will be a way to keep you moving forward successfully. You may be looking to jazz up your current routine or find some new ways to approach your overall healthy lifestyle. You would benefit the most from reading this book in its entirety and taking notes along the way of ideas and strategies that you would like to incorporate into your lifestyle.
- **Maintenance:** Like those in the action stage, you're already living the healthy lifestyle. You may have a cheat day or off-day here or there, but you've been chugging along successfully. This book can be helpful to you as a tool for keeping things interesting and motivating you to continue living healthfully. I would recommend that you thumb through and read the pillars that look interesting to you and that you think could enhance your lifestyle.

Declare Your Independence

Declare your independence from one-size-fits-all programs, misguided advice, and the world's expectations! Using your results from the assessments in this section, examine yourself in an accepting and non-judgmental way. Simply be curious about yourself. If you need to, talk out, journal about, or think through anything that is a sticking point for you. Maybe you've discovered unresolved issues or emotions. Maybe you have some reservations about making changes. Let it out and work through everything. This isn't something to speed through since any unresolved emotions, beliefs, or issues will affect your success and what you can achieve.

Now that you have a better idea of where you stand with your values, beliefs, and attitudes, take a deep breath in, and then, along with all of your past behaviors and negativity, let it out.

You are the creator of your own health, the designer of your happiness. Use this information on your values, beliefs, and attitudes to decide what is necessary for your success, and write a list of the takeaways. Focus on the positive. These important nuggets may be what you're good at, where you excel, what is important to you, reasons for wanting to change, or what your potential barriers to success could be.

Now that you know more about yourself, we're going to build on this knowledge in the second pillar, Goal Setting, to formulate your perfect plan.

PILLAR TWO: GOAL SETTING

Diana Scharf Hunt said, "Goals are dreams with deadlines." This is true in my experience, and it's good news, too! Hunt shows us that our dreams can absolutely be realities—if we plan them out. Goals are necessary for self-improvement, progression in work and life, and in relationships. Goals generate effort and help us to direct our attention, focus, and actions to spending our time on the key strategies and tactics that will make our dreams reality. They also keep us from wasting time on what is either too much work for too little payoff or what is total fluff that doesn't help us achieve our desires.

Using the skills you learn in this book, you can develop a goal mentality that will help you accomplish tasks in all areas. Goals are self-fueling: the more you pursue them and accomplish them, the more you'll be able to do. Think of it like a success workout that provides the same benefits and returns of a physical workout.

To make this healthy lifestyle you're working toward easier and easier, you'll need to learn how to be good at setting, working toward, and achieving goals. You need to work on:

motivation, commitment, determination, persistence, and discipline. These qualities aren't the whole story, though. You're not a goal-achieving robot. None of these alone will get you to that success point, and this isn't to say that you need to use all of these qualities at once or at your full capacity all of the time to achieve goals. You will tap into each one at different times.

In the beginning, you'll mostly depend on motivation and commitment. You'll be excited to start on the road to reaching your goals. Eventually, the tasks will seem less exciting or they will get harder to perform. This is when you will need your determination and persistence. Discipline is for those tough times as you are beginning to turn these goal-seeking behaviors into habits. Once you've formed and set your habits, discipline will be less of an issue since you'll be on auto-pilot with your habits.

Ensuring Plan Success

Early in my career, I worked with a client who was a fly-by-the-seat-of-her-pants type. This worked in her professional life as an artist who worked best with little structure and flexibility. Unfortunately, when it came to reaching her health-related goals, it was her downfall. She could never quite articulate what she wanted to do or why, beyond "get healthier" and "do better with food." It was like she was afraid of commitment when it came to what she was working toward! By being unable to nail down her goals, she ended up drifting and not ever feeling particularly committed to anything we worked on.

Luckily, I learned a lesson from that early career blunder. I no longer allow my clients to start programs without deciding exactly what they want to accomplish and why. Sure, it takes a lot of work up front to get those goals to the point of being helpful guides, but doing so helps you know where you are going, what might trip you up along the way, and when you might arrive at your destination.

My methods are not only based in research, but they pull from the best parts of project management to keep you on-course. We are, in fact, defining and managing Project You. We will be using your responses to the assessments in this pillar to determine the elements of your plan. Our main goal in creating your plan is not only to set achievable and sensible goals, but also to keep our focus on your overall objectives (your motivation for embarking on this journey) while working within your constraints.

This pillar and its worksheets may take you a while to complete. Take your time, and be thorough and detailed. Planning out your path to success now, with fresh motivation, will save you from difficult and tempting situations, setbacks, and, let's be honest, a little laziness, in the future.

Let's now talk about the big picture of what we're doing: making a permanent behavior change so it's easy to live a healthy lifestyle.

What is Behavior Change?

In its simplest terms, behavior is what you do and how you act. Your behavior is an external way of showing your attitudes about your health and yourself as well as what you believe in and value. More completely, your behavior is a product of three factors: motivation, ability, and triggers. So, for you to behave in a certain way, you need to be:

1. sufficiently motivated;
2. able to perform the behavior; and
3. triggered to perform the behavior.

For example, let's say you believe that parking farther away at the grocery store will provide you with more exercise than parking close to the door. You also happen to have the attitude that walking more is beneficial to you and worthwhile. Finally, you not only have on comfortable shoes, but you're feeling well and able enough to walk a bit farther. The only thing left before you park farther away and take some extra steps to the store is seeing a good parking space at the appropriate distance away.

If you're like me, you don't notice yourself going through that whole thought process before saying to yourself, "Self, I think I'm gonna park back here and walk a little farther." This lack of conscious thought before performing a behavior is exactly why it's so hard to change what you do and how you do it. Behaviors are habits that we've established through repetition over time.

The good news is that you can change your behavior. One can, in fact, teach an old dog a new trick ... if said dog is motivated enough to break patterns and create a new habit. This pattern breaking and new habit formation is what we call "behavior change." It's pretty much exactly what it sounds like —changing a behavior, hopefully to something more beneficial to you. More importantly, behavior change is necessary to reduce or eliminate your activities that are not getting you to that effortless healthy lifestyle you're hoping for.

In the following section, you'll identify your current behaviors, decide what you want to change, and create a plan for change. But I won't leave you hanging after making a change! Maintenance is a lifelong job after making changes to your behaviors that lead you to a healthy lifestyle. I'll be sure to leave you with a plan for maintaining the new you and finding new and exciting challenges to better your health long into the future.

Vision

You've figured out your worldview, stage of change, and a whole lot about yourself, but before deciding on what your plan will involve, it is helpful to assess honestly your current lifestyle. This includes all time commitments, free time, patterns, and habits you have.

Now, imagine for a moment your ideal healthy lifestyle. What is it like? How do you feel? How do you look? What is different between your current and ideal lifestyles? What could you change to get closer to the ideal lifestyle? Get a clear picture in your head of how you would like to be living a year from now.

Write down some of your initial thoughts about this ideal healthy lifestyle. Think about what is different between your current real life and your ideal life.

We're going to do a little time travel now. I want you to think about the last time you felt your best, where you looked and felt like a million bucks, and life was good. I want you to picture that version of yourself. Get specific, like what was your favorite outfit, when did you feel awesome?

Now, think about what your natural element was back then. Was it at work? At home? Your happy place? Picture that too. I want you to imagine your past self in that environment and keep imagining that until it's so clear that you feel like you're right there with her.

Now stay with me, because it's going to get a little out there for a moment. I want you to spend some time with past you and chat with her. Would she be proud of where you are now? Would she be surprised? When I need to ground myself or find some motivation for my goals, I spend time with past Kelly. You'd be surprised how clear things can become when you look at your current situation from the viewpoint of your past self and what she would have hoped for.

Write down some of your thoughts about that version of you when you felt your best. Figure out exactly what it was about you and your life back then that made it so good.

Now, let's fill in the gaps between what past you would have wanted and what really happened. We're going to time travel to five years from now.

Imagine your ideal future self. How do you feel? How do you look? What are you wearing? Where do you live? Like with your past self, get really specific about everything so that you can imagine yourself sitting with your future self and having coffee with her. Ask her how she got to this point. What did she change in the last five years so that she looks and feels better than she ever has? Brainstorm with her to figure out exactly what you want and need to do to get there.

Jot down what your ideal self's world was like. How did she get to that point? What would you need to do to turn into her?

Okay, welcome back to the present. Going through those visualization exercises may take some time to get everything crystal clear. I do both of those visualizations frequently to ground myself and find my motivation when I don't feel like getting off the sofa or when I just want to eat until I fall asleep.

Once you have an idea of the best version of yourself and what exactly that looks and feels like, it's time to think about your personal vision for what "you, but better" means to you. Thinking back to your ideal future self, identify the most critical things you'd need to work on to bridge the gap between your current self and that ideal self. This worksheet is also in the free program workbook on my website at www.tsirona.com/ybbbook (see the QR code in the Introduction).

Where do you struggle the most? What might require some extra planning and self-TLC?

Why do you want to make these changes?

Continue to ask yourself "why" for each answer. For example, "I want to fit into my jeans from a few years ago." Why?

"Because I remember feeling really pretty and fashionable when I wore those." Why? "Because I like to get up in the morning and just jump into clothes I know that I'll feel confident and look good in."

Try to get to the core of your goals. What touches you emotionally about those goals?

- How will you feel when you reach your goals?
- What will be better about your life if you achieve your goals?
- What is the hardest part of achieving these goals for you? What could be done to make this easier? Who can help you? What can you do to make things smoother?
- Why haven't you changed or succeeded in long-term change in the past?
- If you woke up tomorrow morning with your goal magically achieved, what would be different for you?

Choosing a Focus for Your Plan

Before you can set your goals and get started on your plan, you need a focus (or two) to define the key areas to spend your resources, such as time, money, effort, and energy. I know you're busy and have a ton of demands on you, so we need to use your resources wisely here. The focus of your plan is essentially what you want to accomplish from doing all of this work.

Think about what you wrote for your personal vision. You may already have a clear direction in mind, like feeling more energetic during the day, fitting into a wedding dress, or running a race. You may have multiple areas you are interested in addressing, but aren't able to prioritize them. Or, you may have come into all of this with a less-than-clear focus. No matter the state of your focus, there are two methods that I like to use for fleshing out my thoughts and beginning to establish goals. Both are visual representations of ideas that can get your potential areas of focus down on paper for your evaluation.

The first method is a bubble sheet. A bubble sheet allows you to see all ideas related to your focus without any order or hierarchy. This is a good place to start if you have multiple ideas for your focus or none at all.

We begin with the overarching (and unspecific) goal you had in mind when picking up this book. Let's use "manage energy" as our overarching goal. Yours may be a play on that like, "get back to how I felt pre-baby" or "feel healthier and more energized." Turn a piece of paper sideways so it is wide and in the landscape layout. This worksheet is also in the free program workbook on my website at www.tsirona.com/ybb-book (see the QR code in the Introduction).

Write your overarching goal across the top. Now, draw circles (bubbles) containing everything you can think of that contributes to the problem you are trying to solve. For example, there are multiple factors that contribute to not having enough energy, some that are under your control and some that aren't: eating nutritious food, exercising, childcare, long work hours, supportive friends, etc. These factors that you've listed are ideas for areas of focus that would be part of your plan for taking care of your overarching goal. After you have listed everything you can think of in your bubbles, take a break for a few minutes. Do something completely unrelated to get your mind off of the task.

Now, come back to the bubble sheet and star, highlight, or otherwise note what stands out to you most as what you'd like to focus on first in your plan. Your method for choosing these can be anything – they are easy to do, they're a challenge for you, they are lingering issues you've always wanted to address, etc. It's all up to you. I happen to like picking what's easiest first so I can get some quick wins, but you may not be motivated by that.

After you have identified a few key areas of focus on your bubble sheet, it's time to get some more paper for the second method: mind mapping. This worksheet is also in the free program workbook on my website at www.tsirona.com/ybb-book (see the QR code in the Introduction).

A mind map takes a central idea and surrounds it with connected branches of associated ideas or parts. Pick one of the things you decided to focus on first in your plan. We'll use this as the central idea. Don't worry, we won't let the other things you chose disappear. We'll take one focus per map to flesh out the first draft of your goals. Like with the bubble sheet, allow yourself the freedom to brainstorm and try out ideas and connections.

In the center of the paper, begin with the first focus. The rest of the map revolves around this one focus. Draw a branch off of this focus and write a word that represents that first element or concept that is related to this. For example, if my mind map is using the focus "daily exercise," I could branch off in different directions with: "10,000 steps daily," "group fitness classes," "walk with friends," and "park farther away." For each of these branches, create sub-branches that stem from them to further expand on your ideas and concepts. For "10,000 steps daily," I could create sub-branches for: "treadmill," "walk around building at lunch," "fitness tracker," and "create a 10,000-steps-a-day challenge with friends." Create sub-branches from these and so on until you're finished.

After you have exhausted your ideas for this focus, move on to any others you wanted to explore and create new mind maps. From your mind map(s), highlight the branches and sub-branches that appeal to you. These are the beginnings of your plan!

Setting Your Goals

Before you can set goals, you need to commit to taking time to decide on exactly what you want. Actually develop a vision of what success looks like. Really get that image ingrained in your mind. Now that you can see what success looks like, ensure that this is a goal that you are strongly interested in achieving. Is it worth the work? Will achieving it be satisfying? If yes, consider whether the goal is achievable. It may be a long shot – and that's fine! – but is it even possible? If your goal checks out, you've found one worth pursuing.

There are three types of goals: process, performance, and outcome. Process goals are those that focus on the path to reaching your overarching goal, like finding and joining a gym or purchasing containers for your weekly meal planning. These goals contribute to the strategy and process of achieving, as the name suggests. Performance goals use behaviors and habits that contribute to your overarching goal as the metrics for achievement, like being able to jog for 10 minutes or eating five servings of vegetables per day. Finally, outcome goals focus on the end result or what success looks like to you. These goals answer the question, "If I complete my process and performance goals, then ____." Outcome goals are the desired results of the work you do in your other goals.

While all three types of goals are important, process and performance goals end up giving you more satisfaction and increase your interest in staying on-plan because they are controllable (you control what you put in your mouth, what you do with your body, and how you live your life); they're also flexible enough for you to change them up, if needed.

Outcome goals can be derailed by many factors. Let's say you're trying to lose weight. If you do all of your process and performance goals as planned, it doesn't guarantee that you will lose 15 pounds by June. It also doesn't counteract weight gain from a surgery or injury during your program. So, while outcome goals are necessary for you to visualize and focus on your target, they are the most susceptible to factors you can't control.

Your process, performance, and outcome goals need to have the 5 Cs:

- Clarity – there is no ambiguity in your goal and you know what is expected
- Complexity – goals should include all aspects needed to achieve the outcome
- Challenge – a goal should be something you are challenged enough by that it will give you satisfaction and the sense of accomplishment when you reach it
- Commitment – there has to be a way to keep yourself accountable to the goal, like tracking methods, rewards or punishments, and other ways of connecting you to staying with the plan
- Continuous feedback – measuring and tracking your performance will provide continual feedback regarding the progress you've made toward your goal

You also need two time frames for your goals:

- Short-term: These are the goals you will begin working on immediately. They can be the mini goals that you break longer-term goals into. These goals usually span a few weeks to a few months.
- Long-term: These goals represent the overall purpose of your plan. They likely include your ultimate goal and your finish line.

For example:

- Short-term: Increase my daily step count to 10,000 steps per day, every day, for three months.
- Short-term: Eliminate potato chips from my diet completely within six weeks.
- Short-term: Walk outside with my sister three days per week for 30 minutes.
- Long-term: Lose six inches around my waist in one year.
- Long-term: Be able to finish a marathon after one year of training.

Setting SMART Goals

We all have a vision of how we want to look, feel, and act. Maybe you wish you were one of those yoga ladies who walks around with a green juice. Maybe you dream of crossing the finish line at a 5k, 10k, or even a marathon! Your vision for your healthy self is as individual as you are. Hopefully you made that vision clearer after mind-mapping and thinking through your personal vision in the last section.

In this section, we're going to take those dreams, visions, and maybe even secret wishes and get really specific about how to turn them into reality. Writer Antoine de Saint-Exupery said, "a goal without a plan is just a wish." We love to spend some time thinking about wishes and playing around with them, but what if you could turn those wishes into reality?

Apart from those dreams, visions, and wishes that are physically unachievable by humans, SMART goal setting, detailed planning, and a system of support and motivation can take you from thinking about getting healthy to living that vision of a healthy you that's floating around in your brain.

It's time to look back at your personal vision that you

completed. Why do you want to work toward a healthy lifestyle? What specific, detailed, emotionally-charged reasons did you write down? This is your vision, your finish line where you are satisfied with yourself and energized. Get in touch with those deep, emotional reasons for your success. What does this success mean for you? How might your daily life change? Surely whatever has captured your imagination here will have enough of an impact on your life that you could see measurable results in your attitude, confidence, or even physical appearance, fitness, or energy. I want you to get such a clear vision of life after success that you can practically touch and feel it.

Now that we have this clear idea of success, what is standing in your way? Something must be, or why else would you deny yourself the joy? Where do you struggle the most in trying to reach this version of you? What might require some extra planning and self-TLC? What needs to change about your attitude, environment, support system, lifestyle, or finances to get you where you want to be?

Let's be real here. If you're saying "lack of motivation," I need you to go deeper. What demotivates you? Do you just plain hate running? Is it out of your way to go to the grocery store instead of ordering delivery? What is the hardest part of staying on the path to success for you?

Don't let yourself get frustrated, apathetic, or even stuck not knowing what to do next. If you had the perfect life for reaching your goal, what would be different from your current situation? Would you have a nanny? A personal chef?

Let's take it down a notch from your happy place. What changes could make this process easier and remove obstacles standing in the way of your motivation and ultimate success? Who can help you? What can you do to make things smoother? Most importantly, why haven't you succeeded in long-term change in the past?

I get it. I gained weight during my last few months of grad school and suddenly didn't recognize myself. I went from petite and energetic to overweight and tired all the time. I had the access and the means to work out and eat well. I had my husband's support and encouragement. I also had the time and flexibility to make a lifestyle change. I also happened to be a health coach and personal trainer for goodness sake! What was the problem? Why did I then hang on to the weight for almost five years after gaining it?

I was embarrassed of my weight, especially when you consider the irony of someone dispensing health advice and conducting health motivation research. My first and biggest barrier was thinking that everyone cared about my weight gain. My imagined scenario was someone saying to another, "Oh, you know Kelly ... she's the chubby one." I wasted a lot of time hiding and worrying over something that most people didn't care about, or if they did, they weren't going to give it any more than a fleeting thought.

My second barrier was that I don't love cooking. It's fine, I'll do it, but I'm not pouring over recipes and getting excited to make dinner. This led to a lot of pizza delivery, grocery store prepared food, and meals out. Though I genuinely enjoy going out to eat, I found that the delivery and prepared food were never very good. They were also expensive! I keep itemized and categorized financials for our spending, and I added up the "Prepared Food/Delivery" costs. I hope you're sitting down for this. We spent well over $17,000 on this stuff in a year. If you're not floored by that, let me put that into perspective. You could buy a brand-new Kia for what we ate in junk.

Beyond those two major barriers, I was unmotivated to do my workout. I told one of my friends one night at the gym while I was talking instead of hitting the treadmill, "Ugh, I hate running." You know what she said? "So don't." I hadn't considered that it was an option not to do something I hated. I would never make a client suffer through a workout she clearly despises. It wasn't even a situation where it got better after a few minutes, or I was glad I did it after it was over. I. Hate. Running. A small tweak, changing my workout from a steady, torturous jog to a mix of sprinting and fast walking, was miraculous. A game changer. Think about it. Do you hate a certain exercise or food? Why torture yourself? Just don't.

When you begin to piece together your goals and plan, be both kind to yourself and realistic. Don't commit to 5:00 am workouts if you're not interested in being a morning person. Don't vow to eat hard boiled eggs if you think they're gross.

What are the most important outcomes of this plan for you? How can you get there in the most painless way possible? The secret to habit-change success is to make it easy. You're going to be actively negotiating with yourself while formulating your goals and plan. Negotiate a deal you can live with and still reach your goals. This worksheet is also in the free program workbook on my website at www.tsirona.com/ybbbook (see the QR code in the Introduction).

As you list your most important outcomes, think of them as your first draft of your goals. These are the outcome goals we discussed in the last section. They are helpful because they help you know your finish line. Break each of the outcome goals down into separate goals that you're invested in achieving. Each one should be distinct and have only one outcome. For example, "I will eat 5 servings of vegetables daily" as opposed to "I will eat better food and drink more water each day." It's still general, but it's a clearer outcome for which you can set process and performance goals.

As you draft these outcome goals, start adding your process goals. Remember, process goals focus on the path to reaching your overarching goal. They are the logistics, and they help with the strategy and process of achieving your outcome goals. This worksheet is also in the free program workbook on my website at www.tsirona.com/ybbbook (see the QR code in the Introduction).

Now think about your performance goals. These use behaviors and habits that contribute to your overarching goal. They are what you actually have to do to be successful and achieve your outcome goals. This worksheet is also in the free program workbook on my website at www.tsirona.com/ybbbook (see the QR code in the Introduction).

Why is it so critical to set goals? Doing so properly will not only give you a finish line to reach, but you will also have motivation and direction as you make progress toward your goals. Having clearly defined and written down goals helps you organize your time, resources, and desires to make the most of your plan. Your goals give you something concrete to shoot for. By knowing the target, you can see progress and take pride in what you're achieving on the way to your goal's completion. Reaching your short-term and mid-term goals will also reinforce that you are on the right track and that you're perfectly capable of achieving the objectives you defined above.

The most effective method for goal setting is the SMART framework. SMART stands for:

- Specific
- Measurable
- Actionable
- Realistic
- Time-bound

Those elements come together to create goals that can be planned and measured and, therefore, lead to success. The more your goals follow this recipe for success, the easier they will be to plan, the clearer you'll be on how you're progressing, and the more motivated you will be since you know what you need to do to be successful. Let's spend a little time on each part of a SMART goal.

The most important part of setting goals is to be **specific**. A specific goal sets the boundaries and helps you know exactly what success looks like. A specific goal lays out exactly what needs to happen and closes the door on ambiguity. For example, let's say you want to eat more vegetables. Okay, exactly how many servings for vegetables? Is that per day? Will you get them in at meals, in a smoothie, during snacks? Pretend that a stranger has been handed your goal without context. Would they know exactly what they should be doing? The more specific you can be, the better you can create a plan and measure your success.

The **measurable** part of a goal answers the question, how will you measure your progress? For example, will you track servings or calories for food? How are you tracking? Will you track minutes, distance, speed for exercise? Will you track meditation sessions or minutes? No matter the goal you are setting, you need to have a way to measure progress. Seeing progress keeps you motivated. Not seeing progress tells you that you need to tweak your plan.

Goals need to be **actionable**. Can you take methodical steps that lead you to success? Could you create a to-do list that eventually leads you to goal completion? The goal needs to be designed so you know what action to take to achieve it.

Though we are translating your dreams, vision, and hopes into actionable goals, your goal needs to be **realistic**. Do you want to work out twice a day for six days a week? Cool. What about your job and commitments? Do you want to fit into a certain size? If one were to take measurements of you at your ideal weight, would you fit within that size's measurement range? Some people have larger frames than will fit in their dream size. Consider also the availability of resources, knowledge, and time you need to be successful. Is this goal something that, though possibly a stretch, can be reached?

Finally, your goals need to be **time-bound**. There has to be a finish line. There has to be a consequence to not achieving the goal. Think about how long you will give yourself to achieve your goals. Is this a near-term goal that you will achieve in a week or month? Your goal may even be a small part of a longer-term goal. For example, your goal now may be to lose three pounds in two weeks. The longer-term goal could be to lose 50 pounds in one year.

Let me give you an example. Instead of setting "go to the gym more" as a goal, it's more effective to make it a SMART goal that is specific, measurable, attainable, relevant, and time-bound. A better goal would be "to spend 30 minutes a day at the gym, four days per week for the next six weeks." This goal now specifies what "go to the gym" means and how it is measured—30-minute increments. It is also attainable, since four 30-minute sessions per week is within the United States Health and Human Services' recommended physical activity guidelines for adults. The goal is relevant, since breaking the gym trips into 30-minute sessions reach the overall objective of going to the gym more. Finally, it's trackable, since you can track the number of minutes and sessions weekly and measure the difference over six weeks. Think of creating SMART goals as writing tiny agreements with yourself that help you set expectations.

When creating your goals, physically write them down. You will need to refer back to them, so don't just keep them in your head. You may set multiple goals but it's more helpful if you keep the goals to a minimum, ideally one-to-three goals, and prioritize them to make near-term progress.

While goals are clear and concrete, they are not set in stone. Goals are meant to be tweaked during this process since you'll be learning more about your own abilities and the other factors that contribute to your success. At the midpoint of this plan, we will reassess and reset any goals that need changes. Before reaching that point, you should still be reviewing your goals on a regular basis to stay on the path and focused on your plan.

List each of your goals and go through the SMART process on all of them. The clearer you can make the goals, the simpler it will be to assign the tactics necessary to achieve them in the next section.

What are the most important outcomes of making a change for you? Be detailed when describing them.

Break the above outcomes down into separate goals. Each one should be distinct and have only one outcome. For example, "I will eat more vegetables daily" as opposed to "I will eat better food and drink more water each day."

Now you're going to refine those goals and make them SMART. Don't stop until your goals are so SMART and clear that you could hand them to a stranger and she'd know exactly what you want to accomplish without you saying a word.

Tactics and Planning

In the last section, I referenced Antoine de Saint-Exupery's quotation, "a goal without a plan is just a wish." This is the part where we will bring those wishes into reality with carefully planned tactics. These tactics will serve as the roadmap to your goal achievement.

Before we get to the tactics, I want you to think about your overall strategy for achieving each of your goals. Think of each goal as a result. For instance, in the old question, "How do you eat an elephant?" The goal is to eat an elephant, so the result is an eaten elephant.

The answer to the question "How do you eat an elephant" is, as we've all heard, "one bite at a time." Those bites are your tactics, the steps you need to take to get the elephant—tail to the tip of the trunk—into your stomach. Bite by bite, decided by your overall strategy, you eat that elephant until that elephant is gone.

We approach all goals in the same manner as the elephant. Some of your goals may even seem as hard as making lunch out of Dumbo. But bite by bite, you can accomplish anything. It simply takes a good SMART goal, a strategy, and the tactics to guide you.

We'll start by listing all of the goals you identified in the last sections. This worksheet is also in the free program workbook on my website at www.tsirona.com/ybbbook (see the QR code in the Introduction).

You might have just one goal, and that's fine. You may also have a long list of goals, and while that's great work, you'll want to pare down your list to a more manageable number of two or three for now. You can tackle those other goals after you achieve the two or three most important ones. Don't give up on what you've listed, just tuck them away.

For each goal, write a one to two sentence strategy. Keep it concise and, well, strategic! Like you did with writing your goals, imagine that you've handed the strategy to someone without context. Could they create a plan to execute the strategy from what you've given them?

After writing a strategy for each goal, list out specific things you'll do to achieve that goal. These are your tactics. Think of everything you can do to execute your strategy. How can you remove obstacles and barriers from your life to make way for goal attainment?

Here's an example: Your goal is to eat five servings of vegetables every day for one month. Because that goal is specific, measurable, actionable, realistic, and time-bound, it's relatively easy to write a plan.

Your strategy could be to add vegetables to your meals by increasing servings in your current recipes and eating vegetable-rich foods for meals and snacks. Your strategy should be reasonable and achievable to you. It's your strategy, after all.

Now comes the fun part—thinking of all of the ways you can use this strategy to reach your goal. Remember, these tactics are things that are easy when taken on their own. Make sure to only list tactics that you would agree to do and that don't impose a burden or hardship. You want to select tactics that are so easy it's silly not to do them. The power comes from the additive effect of doing many of these tactics over time to lead to change, bite by bite.

Now, back to our example. To reach a goal of eating five servings of vegetables a day, what little things could you do to add a serving here and there throughout the day? You could make a smoothie each morning with a serving of spinach mixed in. Pretty painless. You could eat a salad for lunch with 2-3 servings of vegetables or make a pot of vegetable soup with a variety of vegetables in it at the beginning of each week. You could also replace your snacks with cut vegetables and hummus.

At this point, you may be wondering why I haven't just given you a plan to follow to get this over and done with. If that worked, I'd absolutely do it! However, studies have shown that when we can make our own decisions and tailor a plan to our specific needs, we're far more likely to stick to the plan and achieve our goals. That's why it's so important to put a lot of thought into this and think of tactics that can easily fit into your life and will advance you toward your goals. Anything you can think of that would help is fair game for this list. Be creative!

As you start to execute your strategy and add these tactics to your life, you will likely find some that you want to adjust or eliminate. You might also think of more that you could add. The more tactics you have to choose from, the better. It's like having a toolkit at the ready to reach your goals. The final list of tactics needs to be those that you'll actually do without anguish.

Once you have your goals, strategies, and tactics, it's time to plan. Unfortunately, you can't live in a bubble where you only have to focus on reaching your goals. Sorry. To be successful and efficient in achieving your goals, you need to figure out how your new tactics will fit in with your daily routine. What needs to change for you to employ these tactics? Are there things you need to buy? Space you need to make? Schedule shuffling to do? How can you most easily and seamlessly incorporate these tactics into your current life?

As you figure out your new daily routine, you'll have a new list of tactics to use to get life in order. Do your best to get those taken care of as soon as possible. We want to create lasting behavior change and health, not take over your life.

Though most days will be routine, which makes changing your health behaviors simpler, life can also throw you curveballs. Work, school, kids, and friends happen, as do holidays, vacations, and sickness. What can you plan now to keep yourself on track? Take the time to be detailed and create backup plans for the inevitable derailments now. Think of your tactics for these situations so you know immediately what to do when it's time for Plan B.

Some situations to consider for your backup plans are:

- Parties and social events
- Holidays
- Getting sick
- Having time constraints with work or other commitments
- Vacation
- Lack of motivation and needing to get re-energized about your goals
- Other barriers to your success in the past

Setting Milestones

Top entrepreneur and serious proof that habits lead to success, Ramit Sethi, says that "laser focus" and success in reaching our goals comes from giving ourselves constraints and getting "crisp" about our goals rather than thinking in big, general terms (11). Once again, there's the power of small but impactful changes. For example, if I asked you what your goal was when you picked up this book, you might have said "work out more." Sure, that's a great place to start, but there are a lot of ambiguities in that goal. How much more? By when? How will you do it? Why do you want to get more exercise? Creating crisp, laser-focused goals is the only way to achieve what you want to.

This is why it is helpful to break your goals down into their smallest bits in order to come up with a plan that is practically bullet proof. These are the tactics you came up with earlier in this section. If you didn't make itty-bitty, super-doable tactics, take the time to go back and do so. When you know what you need to do each day to reach your goal, the process is less daunting. You can make your lofty, ambitious goals a reality by breaking down the whys, hows, and whats of your plan. These elements will feed your motivation and help you form lasting habits that lead you to your ultimate goal. Before moving on to the Mindset pillar that's just around the corner, I want you to be sure you have the world's most solid plan so you can be successful. We're doing the background work now so you don't have to do it ever again.

Milestones are key in your planning process. They serve as check points on the path of your plan so you know when you've made progress. Milestones define certain phases of your plan that are necessary to reach in order to continue moving on. They can be the same as your short-term goals, or they can even be based on certain times if that is motivational. For example, a milestone could be accomplishing a short-term goal of meditating for 10 minutes every morning. You could also use a time-based milestone like meditating for 10 minutes every morning for two weeks straight.

Milestones represent important points during the process of working on your plan. They represent a sequence of events, habits, or behaviors that incrementally build up to something that creates progress. Oftentimes a milestone marks the start of a new chapter in our lives, like a graduation or a significant birthday. You can use milestones in your plan to mark and celebrate different phases or parts of your plan, too.

Tracking Progress

You've done the work to clearly define your goals, including how you will measure your progress. Regularly tracking your progress toward your goals allows you to see trends, make corrections quickly, and celebrate successes that you might not have seen otherwise. With tracking, you'll be self-monitoring your activities, which means you're observing and recording some aspect of your goal-related behavior. Examples might include calorie intake, number of servings of fruits and vegetables, amount of physical activity, or maybe an outcome of these behaviors, such as your measurements or weight. What exactly you track depends on the measurement part of the SMART goals you set. Studies have shown, time and again, that those who track their progress are more likely to stick to their goals and see the results they want. Tracking moves you closer to your goals because it can produce real-time information for you to review. It also serves as motivation because you can see exactly where your work is translating into positive outcomes. Win-win! There are many ways to track progress, and I'm going to go through a few of them.

Now, you can be low-tech and use a notebook or a spreadsheet, or you can use one of the many great apps out there for tracking. I love MyFitnessPal for tracking my food, weight, and measurements and Fitbit for tracking my activity and sleep. I also keep everything in a spreadsheet because I'm a data nerd, and I like to do forecasts of my success. But you don't need anything fancy to start tracking. Sure, there are endless tools available, but don't let worrying about what to use keep you from starting your new movement plan right away. Just start tracking however is easiest for you.

For nutritional goals, there are many ways to track. Depending on your goals, you could track calories, macronutrients like protein and carbs, servings of produce, hunger (1-10 rating), grams of sugar, and much more. I like MyFitnessPal for this, but you can write in a notebook or spreadsheet or even take pictures of your meals.

If you have activity-based goals, buy an activity tracker. An activity tracker, like a Fitbit, Apple Watch, some heart rate monitors, and other similar products, make it very easy to track your progress. An activity tracker can log things like how many steps you take each day, how much distance you travel, how many calories burned, and more. Some even track your amount and quality of sleep! An activity tracker will make it a lot easier to ensure you're getting enough activity to hit your goals.

If you have fitness-based goals, you might keep track of your heart rate. Intensity is the key to getting the most out of your workouts. An easy way to measure whether your workouts are intense enough is to use a heart rate monitor. These look like a watch and will give you different pieces of information that you can use to track your workout intensity and the progress you're making. You might also want to track your resting heart rate. Seeing your resting heart rate get lower and lower over time will show that you're making more progress towards your fitness goals. Try to measure it first thing in the morning, as it'll naturally get higher during the day. If you don't have a heart rate monitor, don't worry; simply count how many times your heart beats in one minute and note the results. But, if you plan to track during exercise, you'll want a heart rate monitor.

For tracking weight loss progress, we are actually talking about fat loss. Since it's not always easy to get a body fat reading, you'll likely use a combination of weighing yourself and measuring key body parts. It's important to understand that the scale doesn't tell the whole story. Weighing yourself can be a good indicator of progress, but it is only displaying the weight of all that's in and on you. This number includes bones, organs, muscle, water, and clothes in addition to what you're really after: fat. Make sure you use your scale in combination with other tracking methods, like body fat measurement or measuring body parts, like your waist circumference. Scales alone aren't completely accurate, for a few reasons:

- Sometimes your body retains water, which can temporarily add to your weight on the scale
- When we build muscle, we might weigh more but look smaller
- The food we eat on a day-to-day basis can also add to our weight.
- This isn't to knock scales; they can be a helpful and easy way to track change. Just be aware of what you are measuring. Ideally, you'd measure your body fat to track true weight loss progress, but this may not be easy for you to access. Your weight takes fat and muscle into account, but your body fat percentage shows you specifically how much fat you have to lose. To measure your body fat, you'll need to use a tool like calipers, and most personal trainers at your gym would be happy to help you with this. After measuring, you simply compare your measurement

using the tool to a body fat chart. You can also get an accurate reading from DEXA scanning, but this will cost a lot more and isn't a particularly affordable option for tracking progress regularly. As with your weight, try to do it consistently at the same time each day.
- Once you know your scale weight and your body fat percentage, you can work out how much body fat you're losing. Work out your body fat percentage to see how much fat you still have left to lose. For example, if you weigh 170 lbs., and you have 33 percent body fat, simply multiply 170 by 0.33. This shows you actually have 56.1 lbs. of body fat. If this number goes down each week, this shows you're burning fat, even if the scales don't show much progress on their own. Remember, scales are measuring your total weight, including that burrito you ate.

A next best option for measuring body fat is your BMI. This is the measurement doctors will often use, but remember it is only a starting point. There are far more accurate measurements, as BMI doesn't take into account your build (you could be very muscular but show as overweight on this measurement). Still, it's a useful place to start. To calculate your BMI, measure how tall you are, weigh yourself, and then head on over to an online BMI calculator. This is mostly useful as a way to track change rather than focusing on the number itself.

My favorite way of tracking weight loss progress is to measure myself weekly. Taking measurements of specific areas is a great way to see if you're losing fat, and all you need is some measuring tape. To get the best measurements, measure without clothing at the same time of day each week. The tape should be fairly tight resting on your skin. It's helpful if you can find a place on your body parts you'll remember, like a mole or freckle, so you are measuring the same place each time. Depending on your goals and where you carry your weight, you can measure any body parts. The measurements I take are:

- Bust
- Waist
- Low waist (aka the muffin top)
- Left thigh
- Left calf
- Left arm

I chose the left side arbitrarily, but I always stay on that side. You may have a difference between sides of your body because of normal muscle development from dominant use. Pick a body part, side, and place to measure and stick with it.

- If none of these measurements appeal to you, you can always track by how your clothes fit or how you look. If you can't notice the subtle changes in the mirror, take a photo of yourself every week, and start comparing results to a few weeks ago. Those subtle changes all add up. Even a small change can make a big difference to your motivation!
- Finally, for goals that are a bit more subjective, like increasing energy, reducing stress, or changing your mindset, keep some notes in a journal throughout the process to record how you're feeling, what has gone well, and what hasn't. Being able to look back on these notes can help you see more subtle shifts in your frame of mind and ease.

This tracking chart is a starting point for what you'd like to measure and track. You can track anything that fits best with your goals. This worksheet is also in the free program workbook on my website at www.tsirona.com/ybbbook (see the QR code in the Introduction).

	Week 1	Week 2	Week 3	Week 4	Week 5	Week 6
Weight						
Body fat %						
BMI						
Bust						
Waist						
Low waist						
Thigh						
Calf						
Arm						

Accountability

Accountability is a major factor in a plan's effectiveness. Being accountable to yourself or someone else adds not only incentive, but a consistent reminder to stay on track to meeting your goals. Over and over, studies have shown that those who self-monitor their health behaviors are more successful with reaching their health goals than those who do not monitor or do so sporadically. Be honest with your logging and measurement, too. Being able to see an accurate representation of your behavior and your progress will help you continue to fine-tune your goals to meet your overall objectives. Your method for tracking, beyond being consistent and honest, doesn't matter much. You can use an app on your phone, pen and paper, photos, stickers on a chart—anything!

I find that a daily review is useful for staying on track and accountable and keeping my motivation going. Each day, take a few minutes to review how things went well with your plan and goals. If you had a stress-free morning because you planned things out the night before, remind yourself how smart and prepared you were. If you happened to go overboard at lunch but then reigned it back in before inhaling cheesecake, give yourself credit for halting any negative behaviors before they spiraled out of control. Take this time to be objective and identify what worked well, what didn't, and what you might want to change in the future. Small slip-ups aren't a big deal, but they can become big slip-ups if you don't stop to notice them.

Who is on Your Team

Research has shown that, hands down, the most impactful thing you can do to boost your chances of success is to have support from people in your social circle. This is in-person, on the phone, or even strangers on the internet. People who can check in on you, help you, or even do the plan along with you can make a big difference.

Take a moment and determine how you will hold yourself accountable:

- Will you be doing this plan with a partner? Who?
- Are you reporting your progress to someone? Who? In what way? How often?
- Are you rewarding yourself along the way (you should!)? How?

To make health changes like the ones you're planning, it can be helpful to enlist experts. It's not required for you to be successful, but you may want to consider who you could go to if you needed additional support. If you were to assemble a team, I would recommend the following members:

- Your doctor

- Health coach
- Personal trainer
- Dietician
- Counselor

Creating your ideal team to support you, no matter who you decide to have on it, gives you the advantage of approaching your goals with a diverse perspective where each member is the expert so you don't have to be. If you're busy or don't want to spend time searching online for quality health information, you can leverage the expertise and point of view of each member of your team to accomplish your goal.

The Habit Loop

Our daily routines are made up of habits. We easily get caught up in these routines that we don't put much thought into—it's just automatic. That's what we're going to do with your new healthy habits—make them automatic so you don't have to think about them. That's how you'll end up living the healthy lifestyle you want to without having to stress over it.

A habit is essentially a shortcut to a behavior process that would normally take more thinking and attention. Think of how hard it is when you learn a new skill, like a dance routine or knitting. It takes a lot of thought at first. You might make mistakes. You might even overthink it (Who, you?). Through constant repetition, though, we teach ourselves to find small shortcuts in the process to decrease our overall effort. Over time, our brains finally get it and we form a habit.

You can speed up this whole habit-forming process by understanding the habit cycle. This cycle includes having a cue, routine, and reward, and it works like this: There is a cue that triggers you to perform a behavior routine to get a reward. For example, when you come home from work, you always put your keys on the table, pour a glass of white wine, grab a pack of Oreos, and let your dog out. You then start to relax, letting your mind transition from work life to home life. The cue is arriving at home. The routine is keys, wine, Oreos, dog. The reward is a relaxing, calming sensation and the sweet taste of wine and Oreos.

In order to change and understand the habit, we need to interrupt it at the time of the cue and provide a different reward. Here's how to break the routine. You arrive at home like most days, yet this time, you will drop your keys, let your dog out, grab an apple, and go straight to the shower or bath to relax. You are replacing the calm and relaxing sensation of a glass of wine with a warm shower or bath and the sweetness of Oreos with an apple.

Tweaking the routine is as simple as understanding where to break the main cue of the cycle. Start small and change cues that you could easily live without. Don't go for the big wins right away, no matter how tempting. Making small changes like this could seem like they don't matter, but it's the small changes that make the biggest difference over time when you make many of them.

Don't Break the Chain

Remember the habit loop: a cue for a behavior to start, a routine where you do the behavior, and a reward for your behavior. This doesn't just apply to changing habits. It's also key in forming them.

Behaviors without reward just don't become habits in our lives since we don't do things that don't benefit us in some way (even if the benefit is pleasurable but actually detrimental to our health). Humans don't work that way. Your goals and all of their pieces and parts need to lead to the ultimate reward— your vision of yourself. By concentrating on these smaller parts where you are forming the habits needed to be the person you want to be, you'll create a healthy, successful self. But you need some incentive along the way.

Creating this new self is a day-by-day process. Jerry Seinfeld explained his career success to aspiring comedian, Brad Isaac, with a story about his daily task tracking and habit formation: "[Seinfeld] told me to get a big wall calendar that has a whole year on one page and hang it on a prominent wall. The next step was to get a big red magic marker. He said for each day that I do my task of writing, I get to put a big red X over that day. 'After a few days you'll have a chain. Just keep at it and the chain will grow longer every day. You'll like seeing that chain, especially when you get a few weeks under your belt. Your only job next is not to break the chain. Don't break the chain.'" Like Seinfeld advised, changing your behavior and getting to that bright, beautiful vision of you is about the cumulative effect of your habits. Bit by bit, day by day, you're creating your new, improved self. It doesn't happen overnight (sadly), but it does happen.

But what if you do break the chain? It's okay! Get right back on the proverbial horse and restart the chain. The overall visual should be a calendar filled with those red Xs rather than focusing in on the blank days where you had a hiccup.

Determining Success

Most of how you determine success for your plan will be based on reaching your goals and the milestones you've chosen. You will likely find some surprise successes along the way that you didn't set as goals or milestones. For example, if your goal is to include nine servings of fruits or vegetables in your daily diet at least five times a week, you may notice some changes before you've made it to your nine serving/five days a week goal. One change may be finding a new fruit that you love. Or, you may have piqued your daughter's interest in eating more fruits and vegetables while trying to make the change for yourself. It will be important to notice the small successes that pop out along the way.

You may also find tactics that work better than others, or that you reach a goal much sooner than expected. You might also find some goals and tactics are total stinkers and decide not to use them again. This is an experiment. There is no right or wrong way to go about this. It's your life, your plan, and anything can be changed. I would like you to focus on keeping your mindset positive and on your accomplishments rather than what has gone wrong. We'll discuss how you can do this and other topics on mindset in the next pillar.

PILLAR THREE: MINDSET

The Messages Surrounding You

Every day and everywhere we go, we're surrounded by messages about our bodies and how to change or maintain them. Magazines and their online content continue to be a popular source of lifestyle and health information for women, so I conducted a study of popular women's magazine articles and advertisements to figure out what weight loss, fitness, diet, and wellness messages women are barraged by. I reviewed magazines with consistently high circulation numbers that cover the typical American adult female population. As a magazine reader myself, what I found wasn't astonishing, but it was sobering.

In the general interest magazines that discuss lifestyle and relationships, like *Cosmopolitan*, *Glamour*, and *Good Housekeeping*, there was a significant number of articles about weight loss, including success stories, tips, motivation, how-tos, common myths, and ideas for getting more physical activity. There's nothing wrong with this, of course. We're interested, right? The tips tended to be sound advice written by or in association with an actual health professional. What was most noticeable was the sheer number of these articles on weight loss in magazines that also featured recipes, fashion spreads, travel articles, and sex and relationship tips.

In addition to the crazy amount of weight loss articles, weight loss-related advertisements were everywhere in these magazines. There were ads for tennis shoes, fitness fashion, weight loss drugs, diet foods, and diet plans. Other advertisements attempted to make the product on the page look "healthy" by promoting characteristics such as health benefits, low calorie/low fat solutions, added vitamins and minerals, and wholesomeness. Unlike the articles, which at least had some sense of science-based information and reality, the advertisements focused on unrealistic, and oftentimes utterly impossible, ways to indulge in the treats you enjoy without guilt.

We're inundated with messages that make us feel guilty about this or that. It's exhausting! Focus on our bodies, don't focus on our bodies, strong is sexy, get skinny in three days, "be bad" by eating dessert, do this diet to be thin, but be body positive and healthy at every size. The messages are confusing and stress-inducing. It makes me want to scream!

The close relatives of the ads that encourage us to indulge in the food we love without guilt are messages that promote products as some righteous solution, or at least a quick one. We see ads that show a product that is "good" for us—like gluten-free muffins—and the longstanding (but ever-evolving) fast fixes, such as diet pills. Overall, the most common messages perpetuate the false impression that there is an easy way to be well, whether through completely nutrient-void diet treats, pills, or fortified "frankenfoods" that promise health and indulgence. It's gross all around.

You're a smart woman. I can tell by the way you're holding this book. Though these messages are everywhere, I won't let you fall into any traps that attempt to ensnare you. The remainder of this book is all about getting you the quality information you need to set up a plan that is tailored to your needs and is based in science, medicine, research, and reality. You're not dieting. You're not depriving, challenging, hustling. That stuff isn't sustainable. It can also make your mindset all kinds of messed up, making life even harder.

Avoiding Perfectionism

Speaking of making life harder than it needs to be, are you a perfectionist? There's nothing wrong with wanting things in your life just so and wanting to work hard to achieve big goals. I'm right there with you. Fellow "Type A" checking in. What's important for us to get straight here is that there is no such thing as perfect. There is also no right or wrong way to go about what we're doing in this book.

Having high standards for yourself is great, but it's necessary to learn to allow for small imperfections. These high standards are not the problem—it's a perception of perfection being necessary for your success or for you to feel like you and your efforts are worthwhile. You're a capable woman and a total overachiever, so If you put pressure on yourself to achieve perfection, you're probably going to get perfection. Unfortunately, you're going to get perfection in only the area on which you're focused, and you'll sacrifice your health and sanity for it.

I'd like you to view what we're doing here as an experiment. The whole point of setting goals, making a plan, and trying it out is to see what works and what doesn't. I'm not expecting you to get it right the first time, and you shouldn't expect that of yourself, either. Even if you're really that good, the chances are next to none that you'll get everything exactly right and won't need to adjust anything in your plan. That may have been more possible if we were doing a rigid, short-term blitz where you have only a few foods, workouts, and ways to live to choose from. By the nature of what we're trying to accomplish—help you live a healthy lifestyle forever after—there will be adjustments, flexibility, experiments, and the need for you to be open to not being perfect. Practicing the following tips can help you avoid falling into the perfectionism cycle as you work through your plan and get to where your healthy lifestyle comes naturally:

- Embrace mistakes and use them as a teaching tool. Knowing what doesn't work is just as valuable as knowing what does.
- Get rid of the all-or-nothing approach.
- Focus on the journey, as that's what you're using to work through your plan. Outcomes matter, but so does how you got there.
- Stop comparing yourself to others. Just like there is no right or wrong way to approach your health goals, no one person has it right or deserves your envy.
- Congratulate yourself on small and big accomplishments and don't dwell on the experiments that don't work out.
- Overall, be kind to yourself; judge yourself and your performance like you would a friend.

You're Right Where You Need to Be

Guess what? Your big honking brain, your overachieving mentality, and your skills have gotten you to this great place in life. We're not eliminating who you are in this program—we're using everything you are as a way to live a healthy and happy lifestyle. For example, I've learned how to use my anxiety like a superpower and have turned my feelings of never accomplishing enough into fuel for making my life how I want it to be.

No matter what you think your downfall is, when it comes to living your healthiest lifestyle, we can find a way to turn it into an asset. We're going to harness your powers for your success in this program.

I'd like you to free write all the things you do well. Big, small, medium—current or as a little kid. Get out everything that you absolutely nail in life. This worksheet is also in the free program workbook on my website at www.tsirona.com/ybbbook (see the QR code in the Introduction).

Super Power Converter

List the attributes, traits, or behaviors you think hold you back. For example, being a perfectionist or losing interest in things quickly. Then, think of how you can use each to your advantage instead. This worksheet is also in the free program workbook on my website at www.tsirona.com/ybbbook (see the QR code in the Introduction).

Example Flaw: I lose interest in things quickly.

Example Super Power Conversion: I am dynamic and open to finding what works and ditching what doesn't. I keep things fresh.

Baby Steps

Did you know that only eight percent of people reach their goals? That's right! The other 92 percent fail within weeks or months. You're going to be in that eight percent because what differentiates the two groups comes down to one simple thing: setting specific and challenging goals like you did in the Goal Setting pillar.

I know you're probably excited to get going on reaching

your goals and you're getting antsy while reading the Mindset pillar before all of the action. I'd like you to go against your nature and slow down. We're going to go slow and think small now to go fast and achieve big later. The truth is, what you need to do is to think big *in detail*. It's necessary to have detailed information, plans, knowledge, and skills for your big goals to become a reality.

It may also come as a surprise to you that we're not overhauling everything in your life. You might be a lot like me and tend toward the all-or-nothing way of addressing things in life. You want to try yoga, so you buy all possible gear and six months of unlimited classes at a studio. You do it for a week and hate it. You abandon yoga completely and feel guilty for doing so. Then you think you'll start meal planning, so you buy cookbooks, save half of Pinterest, and buy containers and gadgets. You prep for one week, but throw out all of the food in favor of pizza and Pad Thai by Wednesday. Then you feel bad about it all.

It's fun to jump in with both feet, but it also leads to a greater likelihood of failure. I'll probably show my age here, but one of my favorite movies as a kid was the movie *What About Bob?* If you've seen it, you might remember Bill Murray making his way through the movie muttering his therapist's advice, "Baby steps, baby steps." Baby steps are the key to making a lasting difference. Dramatic changes are also traumatic changes, and soon enough, we all fall back into the same old patterns we had before. The way to change your health isn't in some grand gesture. Chances are you've already found that out and you recognize yourself in my description of the failed yogi or meal planner.

The way to make a lasting change is with a lot of small steps. The first thing you need to realize is that there isn't a prescribable formula to creating a new you. There are as many ways to achieve results as there are people in the world. I'm going to outline some changes that will get your mind in the right place to create the new you. These changes I'm asking you to focus on may not seem directly relevant to your health goals, but they are critical for creating a mental environment where you'll make lasting change and reach your goals sooner. Let's take a look at the baby steps I'd like you to try.

First, forgive yourself for everything that's happened before this moment. You've tried, you've messed up. Sometimes you succeeded. Somehow it worked out for you, since you're here breathing and reading this. There's nothing you can do about the past. Start fresh and permit yourself not to dwell on what's come before. This might be the hardest part if you're analytical and a bit of a perfectionist. I want you to keep working at it until you truly allow yourself to start fresh now. Nothing up to now matters beyond being data for what does and doesn't work for you.

Next, find out what you want and tell yourself you're going to get it. Like, out loud. The movies like to show people giving themselves pep talks in the mirror. Usually, we're supposed to laugh at that particular scene, but it's an effective strategy. Be bold and be specific. Tell yourself, "I HAVE THIS!" Even if you laugh at yourself while you do it, I want you to hype yourself up.

Your next baby step comes from an old military adage: the only wrong decision is not to make one. Now is not the time to vacillate and be unsure of your goal. Today is your day to make clear, concise decisions. What is the one small positive decision or change you can make today to reach your goal? Today you're going to decide to do it—and then follow through. Don't go Extreme Makeover: You Edition. Just one small thing at a time!

Now, I know you have baggage—everyone does. But there's another type you may not have considered, and that's physical clutter. Why does that matter in a health plan? Clutter causes stress, for one. Also, you're starting fresh and have chosen not to be the person you were before starting this program. So get rid of anything you haven't even touched in a year. You don't need it. That also goes for anything you have around the house that makes you feel bad. Don't keep the stuff you bought when you were gung-ho about creating a home gym and then forgot. It's time to clear that stuff out too!

Track your day. So many women are exhausted and overworked. Find out why by knowing how much time was spent doing what. If there are four hours each day in front of the TV, that might be a place to start, depending on the goals you have in mind. But again, DO NOT change who you are because others insist that you must. I love TV and Netflix! I'm not changing that at all. Make the changes that benefit you personally. Remember, small changes and baby steps. This is not an opportunity to find more things to cram into your life.

Here's a fun one—I want you to laugh every day. You may have to search out something to laugh at, but make sure you do. Make a plan to laugh at least once a day. Make faces at your dog, do something silly, spend time making a child laugh. Laughter will always come back to you in a good way. It's also what cat videos on YouTube are for.

Next, I want you to be like Elsa in the movie *Frozen* and let it go. Let go of what exactly? Anything that makes you mad, is irritating, and doesn't need to be in your life. Easier said than done, but keep in mind that when you are insulted or belittled or treated in a way that makes your blood boil for a little payback, it's already happened. Remember a time when you were hurtful and petty and the way it tore you up inside. Let it go. Consciously tell yourself that this is over. Take back the time you've spent being stressed and mad and maybe replace it with laughter.

Face one fear. Just a little one. We don't need you to cure your fear of public speaking. You can face a fear by getting a little out of your comfort zone. Try a vegetable that looks unusual. Go to a new group fitness class. Close your eyes and just be still.

Keep taking baby steps. The chance to be bold comes every day. The good news is, if you miss one, another will come along soon enough. Try again tomorrow. Remember to permit yourself to be imperfect and to experiment. Combine that with the ability to laugh at yourself, and you will have created a fresh and exciting new you who's ready to nail this whole healthy lifestyle thing.

Embrace the Process

What did you choose to do today? How did you spend your time? Each day, we're all faced with a ton of choices on how to spend our time. What we decide to do largely makes up our lives. In a very real sense, what we eat, how we relax, and the pursuits we consider important decide who we are and what type of life we lead. In addition, our specific and personal decisions make up our world.

Why do any of us choose what we choose? Sure, some things we choose to do seem out of our control. For example, eating, working, and sleeping all appear to be mandatory and, to some extent, they are. Other choices seem to be purely voluntary. Meditating instead of watching TV or spending time doing something that makes us happy instead of mindlessly scrolling through Instagram are examples of this.

Yet, I'd like to venture that at some level, not eating and not letting yourself relax are just as bad in the long run. Sure, if you don't eat, you will die and if you don't take time to unwind you won't . . . at least not right away. However, is that really what's going on? Is the difference between the two choices that different?

What if you ate potato chips and cupcakes every day? Would you survive? I mean, yeah, in the short term, of course you would. You would most likely survive for a very long time before the consequences of your choice to eat poorly caught up with you. Now, what if you never decided to give yourself room to breathe and calm down. Would you survive? Again, of course you would. You would likely survive as long as the person with poor dietary choices would. However, just like the person with bad eating habits, there would come a time when the consequences of your choices would become apparent.

One set of choices leads to poor physical health. The other set of choices leads to poor mental and emotional health and eventually problems with your physical health, too. In both cases, the result is a poorer quality of life. We all should be striving for the highest possible quality of life that we can. After all, as far as we know, we only have one life to live and what the heck have we put in all this work for at school, work, at home, and on ourselves? Don't we have an obligation to make that life as rich and full as possible?

That's what this program is for. We're focusing on all of you —physical, emotional, mental—the whole shebang. This is because a healthy lifestyle is about having everything in balance and feeling a sense of ease. As you progress through this program, it might take you six weeks or six months. Who cares?! All I want is for you to be making steady progress toward your goals. Timing doesn't matter. I want you to let go of timing expectations too. Even the time-bound part of your SMART goals is just a guess. I want you to think of this program and the changes you're making in it as an experiment. Everyone is different, so there is no right way to be healthy. You may find as we go along that you learn things about your likes, dislikes, and what works for you. And that's all that matters here—what works for you.

It's cliché, but you know a journey begins with a single step. We've all heard that, right? Well, it is true that to get to a destination, you should be moving towards where you want to go. A goal without movement is simply a wish, and wishes, unless you have a genie, do not have the power to change anything. So yes, start your journey towards your goal by taking that all-important first step. After all, nothing ventured, nothing gained.

But, there is a problem with focusing solely on the end of the journey. When you focus entirely on endings while at the beginning, you tend to focus all your energy on the outcome goal and not how you'll get to it. By focusing solely on reaching the end goal, you can lose sight of some fairly important things that will happen along the way. Some of these things are so important that they can actually help you reach the destination you set out for. This is what I mean by being open to experimentation. You'll have a lot of surprises as we work through all of this. You may go from being someone who hates to cook to someone with a new cooking hobby.

I want you to keep your eyes open along the way from start to your completed goal. You want to catch what works and what doesn't early on so you can tweak it. I promise you that it's all worth it. Paying attention to what is happening as you change and using that as your motivation to keep going is the difference between a temporary quick fix that you give up in a few months and an actual healthy lifestyle change.

Developing a Goal-Achievement Attitude

Your mindset, beliefs, and feelings all work together to create your attitude, and your attitude can make or break your success with your plan. In this section, we're focusing on channeling the right mindset for success. You may be tempted to skip over this section to "get to the action," but please resist the temptation. Having your mind in the right place is critical for making lasting changes—ones you won't have to keep doing again and again.

Our first stop in creating a mindset that will get you where you want to be is to create a goal-achievement attitude. This is a positive attitude about your goals that can propel you forward toward success.

Let's work a few questions so you can see where you're starting. This worksheet is also in the free program workbook on my website at www.tsirona.com/ybbbook (see the QR code in the Introduction).

1. How might your attitude hinder your success? What do you feel, think, and believe that may prevent you from achieving your objectives?
2. How could your attitude empower you?
3. Do you feel that your prevailing attitude is helping you or limiting you? Why?
4. What's your attitude about your goals? Do you feel positive, hopeful, wary, negative...?
5. What can you tell yourself to help you achieve these goals?
6. What are some steps you can take to get control of your attitude when the going gets tough?
7. Create an affirmation that will help you work toward your goals. For example, "I am strong, smart, and capable of anything I work toward."

In addition to a goal-achievement attitude, it will serve you well to adopt a growth mindset. This term is way overused in the leadership and business world, but it's still an important concept. Let's look at this as compared to the opposite mindset, a fixed mindset. When you have a fixed mindset, you assume that a person's traits, intelligence, and personality are static and can't be changed in any meaningful way. If you succeed at something, it's because of who you are and have always been. It would, essentially, make reading this book pointless.

A growth mindset, on the other hand, is all about one's ability to learn, grow, develop, and change behavior. It's what the self-help and personal development industries are built on. This means that we are in control of who we are and what we can do, and we can improve ourselves if we wish. I'd like you to adopt this mindset and believe in your ability to take control of your life and health. You've already proven that you can achieve tough things in the rest of your life, so why not your health?

The final part of having a goal-achieving attitude is putting aside limiting beliefs, even if they seem extremely real and unmovable. Limiting beliefs are the beliefs that constrain and inhibit us from growing and developing into better versions of ourselves. They are usually beliefs we have about ourselves and our abilities, but they can also be about our circumstances and world around us.

We develop these limiting beliefs over the course of our lives through our experiences and education, and they can result from our fears, excuses, and faulty logic. These limiting beliefs often disguise themselves as beliefs that keep us safe from harm, failure, or embarrassment. Because of this, they are hard to distinguish from helpful beliefs and we tend to go with them because we're better safe than sorry—or embarrassed.

Here is a big, fat list of common limiting beliefs to look out for and try to get rid of so you can grow and achieve your goals:

- I'm not somebody who follows through
- I'm good at starting projects, but I can't finish them
- I'm not worth it
- I don't deserve _____
- I don't have time
- People will judge me
- If I succeed, I won't be able to sustain it
- I don't have the skills
- I don't know enough

- I'm not going to be successful so there's no point in trying
- I'm too old
- I'm too young
- I'm a quitter; I don't finish things
- I'm lazy
- People like me don't _____
- I'll look foolish
- I've tried it before and failed, so I'll fail if I try again
- I can't because I have kids
- I always avoid pursuing goals that matter to me
- What is meant to be will happen
- I don't/wouldn't know where to start
- I don't have the willpower
- I'm just not motivated
- There is no point
- I don't have enough money
- I don't have enough support
- I'm too scared
- I don't know what I want
- Now is not the time
- It's too late to change
- I have too many responsibilities
- I have no clue where to start
- I'm too _____
- I don't have enough _____
- I'm not _____
- I'm just such a _____
- I'm not the type to be self-motivated
- I should be farther along by now
- If I get my hopes up, I'll just be disappointed
- It has never worked before
- I can't get organized
- I've never been able to manage my time well

- I'll never be happy until that other person changes (spouse, parent, child, ex, friend...)
- It's selfish to put my own needs before those of my family and friends
- Nothing ever really changes
- It's better to be safe than sorry
- I don't deserve to be happy because I'm not really a good person
- I'm a terrible cook
- Life is hard
- And the big one: I can't

When you come across one of your limited beliefs (we all have them), ask yourself if it's true. Keep building evidence against it until the limiting belief seems ridiculous and you can let it go or counteract it with reality when it comes up.

Self-Reflection and Visualization

Self-reflection has to do with how you feel about yourself, others, and life. As opposed to just casual thinking, self-reflection is about making a conscious effort to think deeply and allow insights to emerge. This may seem difficult at first—maybe because it feels pointless, or you don't have the time, or you are a little afraid of what you may unearth in the process. The prompts below will help you with beginning a self-reflection practice. You can certainly come up with your own questions for yourself beyond these!

You may want to write out your thoughts, speak them aloud, or just think through them in your head as a meditative practice. Your way of doing this is up to you, and you can do it differently depending on your mood. In your self-reflection time, you will attempt to tap into your subconscious mind where your self-image lives. Your subconscious is the core of your identity and self, and your deeper qualities, like beliefs, attitudes, values, and major experiences reside here, too.

The purpose of this inward exploration is to ask yourself questions about the best subject: you. Make sure you are being a good interviewer to yourself. Don't cut off your thoughts in this process or avoid the juicy topics. Reveal all you can about yourself. Give some of these prompts a try:

- If I could talk to my younger self, I would tell her...
- Make a list of 20 things you can do that you are proud of. These can be talents, party tricks, or even as simple as things you're good at, like making soufflés that never fall.
- Identify a moment where you were overwhelmed in life, but you pulled through and succeeded?
- Make a list of the people in your life who support and love you. What types of support do they provide you?
- What do you love about yourself physically?
- What do you love about yourself on the inside?
- If my body could talk, it would say...
- What do you love about your life?
- Describe yourself in two sentences.
- I feel most energized when...
- Write a list of everything that inspires you — no limits here.
- Make a list of everything you'd like to say no to.
- Make a list of everything you'd like to say yes to.
- How can someone encourage you to succeed in this program?
- What would need to change to make your life exactly what you want it to be?
- What qualities do you admire in people you know? Be specific.

While self-reflection is a journey inward to meet yourself, visualization is an effort to imagine yourself as you would like to see her. Remember the visualization exercises we did in the last section when you visited your past and future selves? We did that not only to get you inspired, but also because visualizing outcomes of your goals or different efforts or situations lets you metaphorically try on possible realities. The most important outcome to visualize is who you hope to see in the mirror after accomplishing your goals. Does she look happy and healthy? Is she smiling? Is she with anyone else?

Professional athletes have been using visualization successfully for decades. They've been able to increase their confidence and improve their performances using techniques that let them picture what success looks like and mentally rehearse each step to get there. Along with enhancing motivation and confidence, using visualization techniques can activate many of the same neural networks as doing the activity itself. If it's good enough for Olympians Michael Phelps and Simone Biles, it's good enough for us!

Of course, visualization isn't magic. You will still have to put in work and be consistent with your efforts to achieve your goals. Visualization is great for keeping up your motivation and helping you stay the course while you do the work. It's also a nice way to meditate.

To visualize effectively, you need to involve all of your senses. This isn't just for those initial visualizations for setting your goals. This is anytime you're using visualization to reconnect and center yourself. When you visualize, pay attention to what you are feeling, hearing, seeing, smelling, and maybe even tasting. You should feel as if you are right there in the vision. Speaking of being right there in the vision, it's important that you are visualizing through your own eyes. If you visualize like a spectator, you'll miss the connections you will make when imaging the outcome from your own perspective. I find this takes a lot of practice, so you may not master visualizing through your own eyes right away.

When you create your vision with your senses fully engaged from your own point of view, make sure the scenes are positive and that they include all steps between where you are and the successful outcome. Go through everything like it's the best you've ever done. Imagine yourself enjoying a healthy dinner while out with friends instead of imagining yourself passing up on the fried foods and desserts. Really focus on each step where you sit down, open the menu, find the option, order it, see it arrive, and smell and see how good it will be. Picture yourself eating it and imagine it tasting delicious and being nutritious. Imagine the conversations you're having with friends while enjoying your healthy meal. Keep going until you finish, pay the check, and leave feeling satisfied.

In addition to visualizing all the steps, really feel and savor the results of what you are visualizing. How does it feel to have a satisfying healthy dinner? What would you look and feel like if you always chose that? How would it feel after you completed a workout? How will it look when you can wear a new outfit that makes you feel beautiful and proud of your progress?

You know what you want to see from yourself. Doing this effectively isn't about wishful thinking or seeing brief moments of success. Seeing this success—really seeing it, feeling it, and knowing it—will increase the likelihood of you realizing that vision and enjoying the results in your real life. Use your big ol' brain to its full potential!

Setting Yourself Up for Success

When tackling big goals, I've said it's helpful to break them down into smaller pieces that you can take one at a time. There is a mindset reason for this, too. Thaler and Sunstein (12) coined the terms "nudge design," and "choice architects." Their nudge design suggests controlling one's environment to make the healthy and effective options the easy choices. They discovered that relying completely on willpower to achieve goals is a recipe for failure and that willpower is a common misconceived notion. The individual, or "choice architect," is responsible for organizing the context in which they make decisions that relate to their goals. It's her job to create an environment where progress toward her goals becomes the easy, default choice. Each decision represents a small piece of a big goal, so each decision can translate to reaching that goal more easily.

To manipulate and architect your context for making changes, you need to:

1. Make sure your goals have been broken down into the very simplest, smallest actions possible when designing your tactics. Reduce them to their basic steps needed to accomplish them. Make it stupid simple. For example, the goal to "create a meal plan for the week" would break down to: determining what you want to eat, researching recipes, choosing recipes, writing a grocery list, going grocery shopping, preparing food to cook, cooking, and packaging meals for the week. Each step is relatively simple and straightforward, which makes the task less daunting and more manageable. This way relies less on that mythological willpower.
2. Make it incredibly easy to do the steps you've broken your goal into. Make everything so easy that you can do these steps without particularly going out of your way. Let's say your goal is to go to the gym three times a week. Have your clothes with you, water bottle filled, time blocked out, and playlist ready to go.

3. Remove or minimize any barrier that would regularly make doing the steps toward your goal hard. Think ahead, visualize, do whatever you need to do to clear your path to success.

If your new behaviors and habits are going to come together to make a long-term, healthy lifestyle, they need to be convenient and easy for you. That's how we create the healthy lifestyle you want that doesn't require future thought. The more you incorporate the principles of nudge design, the more healthy habits you can slip seamlessly into your life.

Success = Good Habits

As we discussed in the last section, your habits are the behaviors that you repeat so frequently that they require very little energy to do, and they get easier to do over time. Habits tend to be deeply ingrained in our mental processes, which is great if they are positive, but not so much if they are detrimental. Changing habits is rarely an easy or quick process because they are so entrenched in our routine behavior. Changing your habits not only takes time, but also a plan and, more importantly, faith in that plan.

Changing habits requires different levels of energy depending on how easy or hard the associated behaviors are. When a behavior is easy to do, you don't need much motivation to do it. If a behavior is harder, you will need much more motivation to do it. Think of how easy it is to get in your car, turn it on, and pull out. It's nearly automatic. I bet you don't even think of the mechanics of driving anymore. Now, think back to when you were learning to drive. How hard was it to remember to put on your seat belt, turn on the ignition, adjust your mirrors, look all around, put the car in reverse, and then back up without hitting anything? It was really hard! That's why it takes time between getting a learner's permit and a driver's license.

Imagine you're just now getting the learner's permit for the new behaviors and habits you want to adopt to reach your goals. You'll need some practice and time. Motivation? Sure, that's nice too, but relying purely on motivation to keep you going while you practice and ingrain these new habits is risky. Motivation by itself is highly unpredictable, and it can change from moment to moment, depending on how you feel, external effects, and your interest level.

Have you ever started a diet or new exercise program and you've been pumped up to make big changes ... but lose that excitement and motivation in a short time? I think we all have. When the going gets tough, even the tough get unmotivated. The way around this loss of motivation and ultimate abandonment of a new program is to start with simple habits that let you focus on achievable mini goals. The smaller and simpler your adoptive habit is, the better you will be able to make it your own and master it without relying on much of that unreliable motivation. That's why I made you break everything down so much in our Goal Setting pillar.

In his popular TEDx Talk, BJ Fogg described his method which relies on this idea of breaking habits down into simple bits (4). It's a lot like the nudge design we talked about for breaking your goals into achievable mini ones. Fogg notes that behaviors are "interlocking parts of daily life" (1). New behaviors that make up your desired habit should relate to the other behaviors occurring around them. These surrounding behaviors can work as a reminder to engage in your new behavior. You know, those same cues that start off your habit loop. It's easiest to use an existing routine to add your new habit, like standing up when talking on the phone or drinking a half of a bottle of water on your commute. You're already used to talking on the phone and commuting; adding in something else isn't a challenge. With this method, it's also important to find a way to praise yourself and feel good immediately after doing the new behavior—even though it's just a tiny new habit you've added. This will condition you to crave that good feeling and make you more likely to perform that behavior. Reward yourself with positive, congratulatory sayings, like "I did it!" or "Success!" It might feel silly at first, but drawing positive attention to yourself after completing the behavior will give you an emotional surge. Eventually, with repetition and consistency, these behaviors will become your new positive habits and you won't need to rely on motivation.

The Motivation Wave

Motivation ebbs and flows depending on your interest as well as the other things in your life that are competing for your attention, like work, chores, kids, and friends. At the top of your motivational wave, you are engaged and interested in tackling a new habit and in the prime position to set up a system for making changes. You're probably riding that wave right now since you've recently started reading this book. Motivation only has one role in our lives—to help us do hard things. This makes sense since we need little motivation to perform easy habits like showering and brushing our teeth. By building your system for how you will use a series of small habits to lead to a bigger habit change at the top of the motivational wave, you don't have to do much when the motivation is low. If you follow your plan, you won't have to muster up motivation later on; you just do what your plan says, even when motivation is at its lowest point, crashing into a shore of procrastination. At that point, you can still take baby steps and accomplish the tiny, manageable habits you built into your system back when you were motivated.

How do you create a system? Think about the habit cycle. You need a cue that will kick off this itty-bitty new habit as a part of your *existing* routine. We're not creating a whole new routine for this. For example, when you brush your teeth (cue), you add a new habit into the routine of actually brushing—you pace around the bathroom to get in a little more movement.

Once you have an idea of your new system for creating these habits, give that system a test drive for 30 days. I suggest 30 days for two reasons: focus and seizing opportunity. First, you'll be focused for a limited amount of time, and, therefore, will know that there's an end point and days you can track. You can do anything for 30 days! Second, without jumping in and trying out your system while you're excited and motivated, a month could easily pass by without action. It's also a short enough time period to change out the habit at the end if it isn't working and you won't have wasted time once that motivational wave pulls back out to sea.

Rewards

Most of us are motivated by rewards. This doesn't mean unhealthy rewards, like a large pizza and brownies (I tried. . .that didn't work out so great). Instead, choose rewards that mean a lot to you but that won't negate your efforts! There's a saying, "Nothing succeeds like success." This is based on the idea that one success drives you to another. It's invigorating and motivating to have a win. You're anxious to get that next win! Setting goals and milestones like we've done in this program designs a path that guides you to these small wins. Each achievement is a reward in itself, but sometimes you need a little something more.

An effective and fun reward to plan for yourself is something that is of interest to you and dependent on meeting your goal. You can pick material rewards, like a new shirt or earrings, or you can give yourself something intangible but valuable, like a day off from work or a nap. Keep in mind that planning for frequent small rewards that you earn for meeting your milestones are more effective than bigger rewards that require a long, difficult effort to earn them. You're looking for momentum and motivation.

I want you to choose your own rewards because of something called choice bias. You now know that we're more likely to repeat actions that lead to rewards, but this is especially true when we're in charge of the prizes.

Your rewards can be anything but food. We're trying to break the food-as-reward association! Be 100 percent sure your reward won't undermine your efforts. Here are some ideas to start thinking about your own rewards:

- Take a guilt-free nap
- Have a spa day
- Sleep in and have a leisurely morning
- Post your progress on social media so your friends can celebrate with you
- Take a vacation day from work to do whatever you want
- Watch or go to a movie
- Plan a night out with your friends
- Make a new workout playlist
- Get yourself flowers
- Try a fresh hair color or cut
- Buy a pair of high-end headphones
- Invest in a fitness tracker
- Treat yourself to a massage
- Take a cooking class
- Get fitted for workout shoes at a running store

- Plan a weekend getaway
- Hire someone to clean your house
- Schedule a professional portrait shoot
- Get a new item of workout gear

Do not neglect to plan rewards. It may seem like a frivolous part of the plan, but decades of research shows that well-chosen rewards help us stay motivated and establish long-term habits. It's worth your time to come up with a list of rewards for your milestones!

Contract with Yourself

I recommend committing to yourself in writing. This worksheet is also in the free program workbook on my website at www.tsirona.com/ybbbook (see the QR code in the Introduction).

I, _____, hereby agree and commit to take the following steps to improve my accountability to myself and increase my chances for health success:

- I will have faith in my ability to set goals and create a plan to reach them.
- I will trust my plan.
- I will not let one small slip-up convince me that I'm a lost cause.
- I will respect myself by refusing to engage in verbal self-abuse, and I will find positive ways to comfort and support myself when I'm having a hard time. Specifically, I will: [Make a list of concrete things you will do instead of beating up on yourself or deciding your problems are too big to handle.]

When there is a conflict between my plan and what other

people want me to do, I will negotiate to find a reasonable solution that allows me to do what I need to do for myself. I choose to be in charge of my own decisions and behavior.

If I do not comply with the above terms, the following will happen:

[List consequences for not following your contract]

If I succeed in progressing toward my goals, I will reward myself with the following:

Signed,

_____

A MOMENT ON WEIGHT LOSS

Weight Loss in a Nutshell

For over 25 years, more than half of the adult population in the United States has been overweight or obese. Each year, we are seeing more weight problems and more weight-related health issues in our population. The Center for Disease Control and Prevention (CDC) found that 67.4 percent of adult females were overweight or obese (2). This obesity epidemic is only continuing to get worse. As we age, the likelihood of gaining weight and having resulting health problems increases. If that doesn't scare you, get this—rates of hypertension, abnormal blood lipid profiles, and diabetes are higher in adults with abdominal obesity. It's not all about looks. It's about the quality and length of your life!

For decades, American culture has obsessed over being skinny and the ideal body. With this has blossomed a monster of an industry dedicated to weight loss. We read, hear, and see crazy claims for quick fixes or miracles that don't even make sense in the first place. But why do so many people try these quick-fix gimmicks and false-hope traps? They are desperate to solve what they see as the problem rather than a symptom of other problems. Extra body fat is not the problem in itself that needs to be burned, frozen, vibrated, or wished off. Excess body fat is only a symptom of other behavioral and health issues. It doesn't make someone bad or lazy or ugly.

Beyond the obvious snake oil sales claims and tabloid cover ridiculousness about miracle diets, there are some moderately legitimate sounding claims floating around about obesity, being overweight, and the reasoning behind both.

A common trap that many women fall into, especially as they age, is placing blame for excess body fat on metabolism or genetics. Let's start with the metabolism argument. Having a "low" metabolism has very little to do with causing obesity. In fact, as one carries more weight, her metabolism will go up because more energy is expended by a larger person during normal daily activities. Smaller people have lower metabolisms because it requires less energy for activities. Multiple studies over the last 30 years have consistently disproven a connection between resting metabolic rate (your "metabolism") and weight.

Metabolism-wise, what is significant in weight loss and management is your basal metabolic rate (BMR). This is the measure of rate of energy you use when resting to keep vital body functions going, like your organ functions, maintaining body temperature, and breathing. This is what you're burning when you spend all day in bed watching Netflix. Your BMR is determined by a combination of factors, including: age, sex, genetics, and, most importantly, body composition. While you can't do anything about your age, sex, or genetics, you can control your body composition.

Body composition is what you're made up of. There's fat mass (body fat) and fat-free mass (muscle, bone, water, guts, and everything else that's not fat). We tend to measure this by telling you your body fat percentage. You want to have more fat-free mass and less fat, but you do want some fat.

Your body composition doesn't always match up to how you look or what you weigh. If you are hitting the gym hard and you have lower body fat and have built muscle, you'll likely look lean but weigh more than you'd think. There's also what you may have heard called "skinny fat." This describes people who look thin, but who actually have a high percentage of body fat compared to fat-free mass because they are low on muscle tone. You'll want to be somewhere in between. There are the general guidelines for body fat percentages in women—remember, women almost always have more body fat than men, so make sure you're following these guidelines for women:

- Top athletes: 15-20 percent
- Fit women: 21-24 percent
- Healthy/acceptable: 25-32 percent
- Overweight: 33 percent and above

It's important to remember that changes in your BMR come over time and from long-term changes made in your lifestyle that help you add muscle and lose fat. Building muscle while working to lose fat is beneficial because, even when your body is at rest, your lean muscle mass will burn more calories than your fat stores would.

Besides just knowing it exists, what makes BMR a useful tool if you want to lose or maintain weight is that it can be used to calculate a daily calorie intake goal. You can reasonably approximate your BMR with a calculation, as shown below, or receive a more precise number through a laboratory test.

BMR for women = 655 + (4.35 x weight in pounds) + (4.7 x height in inches)—(4.7 x age in years)

Your BMR results are the calories (energy) your body burns at rest. In other words, the amount of energy needed just to keep you alive. This is different for us because our bodies are unique. Do keep in mind that BMR is just an estimation, as your body changes daily. For example, if you are sick or injured, your body will use up more energy to repair and, therefore, would use more calories to do so.

If you are interested in weight loss or maintenance, we will take this calculation a step further by using it to calculate your Total Daily Energy Expenditure (TDEE).

When you do anything beyond just lying there surviving, you burn additional calories. When you combine your BMR with the calories you burn through physical activity of any sort, you get your Total Daily Energy Expenditure.

To figure out your TDEE, multiply your BMR by the appropriate activity factor below:

- Sedentary (little or no exercise): BMR x 1.2
- Lightly active (light exercise/sports 1-3 days per week): BMR x 1.375
- Moderately active (moderate exercise/sports 3-5 days per week): BMR x 1.55
- Very active (hard exercise/sports 6-7 days per week): BMR x 1.725
- Extra active (very hard exercise/sports & physical job or 2x training): BMR x 1.9

Your result is the approximate number of calories you need each day to maintain your weight. Be aware that this isn't an exact calculation, and there are some issues with calorie measurement that are above our pay grade to know. The important thing is to know the ballpark calorie amount.

But what if you want to lose weight? You lose weight by

having a calorie deficit. This means that you either eat less than your TDEE or be more active.

Now, about genetics as a reason for obesity, weight gain, or difficulty losing weight. Yes, genetics play a role in your BMR, but this role is a minor one. Unfortunately, many people are using genetics as a scapegoat for unhealthy behaviors. The human genome's effect on weight has been greatly exaggerated. Why? Because it's easier to place blame on aspects of our lives we have no control over, such as genetic dispositions and certain conditions. The truth is that you are usually in control of a significant part of your health. You have the capability to be as active as possible to your ability and to eat nutritious foods. You are beyond excuses and putting power into things you can't change.

Here's what your genes do influence: the shape of your body. Your long torso, short legs, broad shoulders, and anything else about your skeletal shape is based on genetics. The other parts are on you—and you can be anything you want. According to a Danish study of twins, researchers concluded that the "evidence that genes could affect the proportions of the human body had been overestimated and couldn't explain the increase in obesity [for one twin over the other] over the past 70 years." (5) The researchers suggested that it is the individual's habits that play the most important role in weight. Well then.

I want to bust two myths about how you get to a healthy weight. The first is a carryover from previous decades when the personal fitness craze was just beginning. Most Americans believe that exercise is the key to weight loss and that more time in the gym will lead to more progress. Exercise's health benefits can't be overstated, but exercise is not the best tool for weight loss. The actual percentages are argued, but experts agree that diet is the more significant part of the diet-exercise duo for weight loss.

Your diet, though, doesn't need to be special, brand-name, or expensive. Fad diets are fads for a reason—they don't stand the test of time (or science). There's a common saying in the industry that diets work . . . until they don't. You will probably lose weight on a juice cleanse or a very restrictive low-calorie diet. That's great until you have to maintain that loss. After the initial loss, fad diets pile the pounds back on, and they bring a few additional pounds along with them. We're not doing a diet, per se, in this book. It's about eating healthy, nutritional food most of the time. Your plan will be balanced and maintainable, and it will fit into your lifestyle forever after.

The Focus on Weight as a Measure

Body weight is a helpful measure, but it is not the only effective one. Your weight when you step on the scale is simply a measure of how heavy everything inside you and on you is at that moment. Your weight can be influenced by your hydration, time of day, time of the month, and even your sleep. But, measuring and tracking weight becomes more helpful over time as you can track change, and weight can provide insight alongside other data, like body circumference measurements, food and exercise tracking, and mood tracking.

If your short- and long-term goals include weight loss, they will depend on you making lifestyle changes to affect your weight and size. Long before you see significant changes in your weight, you will feel better overall with increased energy and a positive outlook. This is what will fuel you to reach your weight loss goals in the long term. Remember, your weight is not *who* you are. It's the state of your body as a result of your completely controllable lifestyle.

Your health and your future health are both in your control. You can change your mindset and behaviors starting right now to live a long, healthy life. All it takes is arming yourself with information and formulating a plan you can follow. As Maya Angelou said, "When you know better, you do better." I'll make sure of that in this book. There are two areas we need to know more about to change body composition, movement and nutrition, which we'll discuss in the next two pillars.

PILLAR FOUR: MOVEMENT

Why "Movement"?

In this pillar, I use the term "movement" because it encompasses exercise that is considered either activity or fitness. Don't worry—we will discuss the difference between the two in this pillar. The other, and greater, reason I use movement is to remind you to incorporate moving around, however you prefer, into your daily life instead of waiting to go to the gym and exercise, which can be daunting at first.

Movement Roadblocks

Did you know that even 30 minutes of physical activity on most days can improve your health? It's not even about strenuous exercise or anything hard, just moving. People who exercise regularly are healthier in almost every way than those who don't. That makes sense, right? Here are some of the specific benefits of regular exercise found in the research:

- Reduces the risk of infections
- Eases asthma
- Prevents heart attacks
- Controls blood sugar
- Protects against cancer
- Combats stress
- Relieves hot flashes
- Prolongs life

These might not sound that exciting if you're in your 20s or 30s, but your habits and behavior now directly affect your future health. Exercise keeps you young. Ooh, did I get your attention? When you do workouts that get your heart pumping even a little, oxygen flows through your body and you improve your aerobic capacity. Aerobic capacity is the highest amount of oxygen that your body consumes during your highest level of exercise in activities that use the large muscle groups in the legs, or arms and legs combined. Even a small improvement would be like taking 10-20 years off your age. There's more! Regular exercise is great for your skin, and it creates a beautiful glow. Bottom line, people who exercise regularly are healthier, look better, and age better.

There are lots of roadblocks and reasons people have for not exercising. In my doctoral program, I did a survey of women 25-70 years old to see what they considered their biggest challenge when it came to incorporating exercise into their lifestyle. It was interesting to see the responses. I felt like I wasn't alone, since I've felt all of these! They responded:

- Cost
- Getting started
- Time
- Putting others' needs above their own

- Feeling too self-conscious
- Fear of not being able to stick with it
- Not knowing what exercises to do
- Not feeling motivated to start
- Feeling too tired
- Not liking to exercise

The three most common categories of roadblocks that come up with my clients and in my research are time, knowledge, and motivation. Because all of us are busy, and fitting everything into an already busy schedule is a huge challenge. It's tough not only to find the time to squeeze in exercise, but you also need to figure out what you want to do. Pilates? Crossfit? Treadmill? It's a lot. That's why knowledge is a big roadblock. People may join a gym or want to exercise at home but don't know which exercises or types of activities are best for them. Often, they know what they'd like to do but don't know how to do the exercises properly. Or, they're afraid to try things to see what works.

Finally, there's motivation. We lean on this one a lot as an excuse because we really believe that we just need to muster up the right motivation. You learned in the Mindset pillar that not only does motivation not last, but it's not really enough to keep you going.

Wherever you are right now is your starting point, and that's okay! Start where you are and acknowledge that you are going to move forward from here. Will one workout make a difference? No. Will four workouts make a difference? A little, because you'll get comfortable and in the flow of it. Would 208 workouts make a difference? Heck yeah! If you worked out just four times a week, at the end of a year you would have worked out 208 times! A year from now, imagine how you would feel after 208 workouts. It all comes down to your daily habits.

You might need to experiment a little to find the workouts you like. There's no reason at all to do something you don't enjoy! The workout that your best friend loves may not be the workout you love, and that's okay. I have no rhythm, so if a friend invites me to a Zumba class, it's never going to happen. If, on the other hand, I have a chance to take a kickboxing class or go for a long walk, I'm there! Figure out what you enjoy and what fits your personality and your goals.

Exercise really can be fun. For real. Here are just a few ideas:

- Dancing
- Rowing, kayaking, canoeing
- Biking
- Skating
- Swimming
- Group fitness classes
- DVDs and online workouts
- Yoga
- Pilates
- Kickboxing
- Martial arts
- Boxing
- Stand-up paddleboarding (SUP)
- Hiking

There are so many possibilities other than walking and running. This is by no means a complete list, of course, but maybe it will spark an idea for you. Be adventurous and try something new.

Movement Motivation Self-Assessment

Using my research on exercise barriers, I created an assessment to help find a starting point for movement goals. While setting those goals, I found there are four important parts of getting, and staying, active for women:

- **Goals.** Do you want to feel stronger? Do you want to have more energy? Lower your "numbers" or a specific part of your bloodwork? Do you want to feel more attractive? This area looks into your desires—this is the "what" of your goals.
- **Interests.** Do you like to get outside? Do you prefer structured fitness classes or a personal trainer with a specific plan? Do you want to learn a set of exercises to do at home? This area explores what you want to do in your exercise. If you want to get out and ride bikes with your family, it would be counterproductive to have you in the gym on the treadmill for an hour a day, right?
- **Sources of motivation.** Why are you making these changes? Why do you want to achieve your goals? What do you think is going to change for you if you are able to change? There has to be a good reason behind making a change to keep you moving forward.
- **Barriers.** We all have something standing in the way of our goals, big or small. Once you can identify what is in your way, you can brainstorm ways to remove or get around that barrier. Nothing is impossible with the right plan for the job.

On the following assessment, select responses for each question. After you respond, see the key below each question for tips to help with your exercise plan. If you prefer, you can take this assessment online at www.tsirona.com/FMA.

1. Age Group

- 18-24
- 25-40
- 41-50
- 51-70+

If you are 18-24: You have youth and time on your side. You may be a student or young in your career, which can be stressful. Take advantage of school, club, and local activities; sports; and classes to make exercise fun and social. If money is a factor, you can often find student discounts at local gyms and studios.

If you are 25-40: Women your age tend to be busy, overcommitted, and trying to do it all. Though it may seem there is no room for exercise in your schedule, you are likely to find stress relief and enjoyment in being active. Try different activities until you find what works for you. If you have children or other family members at home with you, include them in your exercise... unless that's your "me time."

If you are 41-50: As life starts to change—kids are growing up, careers are stable—you may find some new opportunities in your schedule for activity. Whether it is gardening, running, swimming, or a fitness class, there are countless ways to get in your exercise. At this point in your life, make sure you are doing strength training to maintain bone density.

If you are 51-70: At your age, you may be transitioning into a new way of life regarding health. While you may be finding that your weight is harder to maintain or that you have less energy than you did in the past, this is still a great time to get your body into great condition and to use the experience and knowledge you've gained over the years. In order to take full advantage of all the benefits of more physical activity, you have to (1) commit yourself to investing in your health wellness as much as you commit yourself to others and (2) use your resources—like fitness websites, a personal trainer, books, fitness classes—to understand how to do specific exercises that will have you feeling healthy for years to come. The reward of being stronger, more flexible, more fit, and glowing from the inside out may be exactly what you need to get, and stay, motivated and energized.

2. Do any of the following special health states apply to you? If not, please continue on to the next question.

- **Disabled/In Significant Pain**
- **Pregnant**
- **Perimenopausal**
- **Menopausal**

If you are Disabled/In Significant Pain: Women with disabilities or chronic pain benefit from including as much activity as they are able to, spread across the week. Be sure to consult your healthcare provider about the types and amounts of activity that are appropriate for you. If you are able to, you should get at least 150 minutes per week (2 hours and 30 minutes) of moderate-intensity aerobic activity performed in episodes of at least 10 minutes, and preferably, it should be spread throughout the week. You should also do muscle-strengthening activities of moderate or high intensity that involve all major muscle groups on two or more days per week, as these activities provide additional health benefits.

If you are Pregnant: Healthy women who are not already highly active or doing vigorous-intensity activity should get at least 150 minutes (2 hours and 30 minutes) of moderate-intensity aerobic activity per week during pregnancy and the postpartum period. Preferably, this activity should be spread throughout the week. If you habitually engage in vigorous-intensity aerobic activity or are highly active, you can continue this physical activity during your pregnancy and the postpartum period, provided that you remain healthy and discuss with your healthcare provider how and when activity should be adjusted over time.

If you are Perimenopausal: Many women start to feel tired as menopause approaches. It may seem counterintuitive, but a bit of activity may be what you need to re-energize. Include a variety of cardio, strength, and flexibility workouts to ease the transition and changes that are coming.

If you are Menopausal: Many women feel tired during menopause. If you need to re-energize, consider getting in some activity. You can do an exercise session or even just go for a walk with the dog. If hot flashes are a problem for you, consider going to the pool for a water aerobics class or a swim. That way, you can stay cool and get an excellent workout! If you think that's for the old folks, think again. When I taught water aerobics, I had classes with women and men from their 20s through their 80s who were in excellent shape.

3. Do you have children at home?

If yes: Any mom knows that chasing the little ones around, cleaning up after the family, and getting everyone ready and where they need to go counts as exercise. Even better, playtime can be family *and* movement time! For those with older children, consider using the time between piano lessons and soccer practice as bonus "you" time to take a walk or stretch or hit the gym with some friends. Making your health a priority is often difficult for women, especially those who are busy caring for others. Take time to care for your own wellness so you can keep up with the kids.

4. Do you work or attend school during regular business hours (9-5)?

- Yes, regular business hours
- No, I have hours outside of those times (e.g., shift work, night shift, late classes, stay-at-home mom)
- No, I don't work or attend school

If you work or attend school during regular business hours: If you have a job where you are seated for most of the day or you spend hours in class, it is especially important that you make sure you are getting up every 30 minutes for a quick stretch or a walk around. Many companies and schools have gyms in the building or nearby—yours may even offer a discount or incentive for joining the gym. You can also gather coworkers or fellow students and create a movement challenge where you are accountable to each other and can provide support and encouragement. In order to put your health first, choose a time of day to exercise that works best in your schedule. Maybe giving yourself an extra half hour in the morning to take a walk or run will make all the difference. Or, you may benefit from keeping a gym bag in your car and hitting the gym on the way home.

If you do not work or attend school during regular business hours: With the availability of 24-hour gyms, DVDs, online fitness classes, and simple at-home fitness activities, your schedule does not need to be a hindrance to getting more activity. Take advantage of your schedule and get in some time at the park, the gym, or the mall when they are less crowded. Any activity, whether it's cleaning, grocery shopping, or dancing in Zumba class can get you stronger, healthier, and happier! However, if you have a job where you are on your feet, you're entitled to some relaxation after work. Instead of sitting in front of TV, wind down with some quiet yoga or stretching.

If you do not work: Well, the world is your oyster! Take advantage of your flexible schedule and get in some time at the park, the gym, or the mall when they are less crowded. Any activity, whether it's cleaning, grocery shopping, or dancing in Zumba class can get you stronger, healthier, and happier!

5. What do you wish you understood better or knew more about when it comes to movement, including fitness, exercise, and being active?

- How to fit physical activity into my schedule
- What exercises to do
- How to do exercises
- Specific benefits of being more physically active

If you want to know how to fit physical activity into your schedule: Sometimes what's standing in the way of you and your workout isn't lack of motivation—rather, it's simply finding the time. Committing to a fitness class, working out with a friend, or getting fit with a personal trainer can keep you accountable. Scheduling exercise can also be helpful if you tend to run out of time. But you won't always have an extra hour for the gym. Scheduling exercise may not be as difficult as you think if you get creative by parking farther away, taking the stairs, walking at lunch time, and taking little movement breaks throughout the day to get your heart pumping for a short amount of time. Even a 2-10 minute bout of activity a few times a day is good!

If you want to know what exercises to do: Cycling, interval training, cardio kickboxing—who can keep track? There are so many ways to be fit and active these days that it can get confusing when all you want is to know how to get great legs or how to run a mile. For advice on the perfect exercises for you and for your goals, set up a consultation with a personal trainer (lots of times it's free), look through fitness websites and magazines, or go with a tried-and-true method—exercise videos. In addition to ones you can buy, there are endless free how-to videos on YouTube and there may even be a selection at your public library.

If you want to know how to do exercises: It can be a waste of time—and potentially harmful—if you try to do exercises without understanding technique. Be sure to clarify how to do movements with a personal trainer or fitness instructor. They can also teach you how to modify exercises to better suit your needs or fit your skill level. Don't be shy if you're new in a group fitness class. Let the instructor know so he or she can keep an eye on you.

If you want to know specific benefits of being more physically active: According to the Mayo Clinic, there are seven important benefits you'll get from increasing your physical activity: (1) control weight, (2) combat health conditions and diseases, (3) improve mood, (4) boost energy, (5) promote better sleep, (6) put the spark back into your sex life, and (7) have fun.

. . .

6. If you had all the time and resources you needed to achieve your personal movement goals, what would those goals be?

- Getting stronger
- Gaining flexibility
- Being more attractive
- Living a longer life
- Getting in better aerobic/cardiovascular shape
- Improving my "numbers" (e.g., cholesterol, blood pressure)
- Preparing for an event (e.g., race, triathlon, competition)

If your goal is getting stronger: Strength training isn't just for beefcakes and strongwomen. Whether you like machines, free weights, or working with your own body weight, there is a strength-training regimen that fits your needs. Be sure to speak with a personal trainer or consult an expert before using new machines or heavier weights than usual. In general, training with high repetitions will allow you to build muscle and get an aerobic workout at the same time. Time saver!

If your goal is gaining flexibility: Flexibility is gained through persistence and continuity. Stretching after workouts and throughout the day will improve your flexibility. Activities such as yoga, Pilates, and dance are fun ways to increase total-body flexibility.

If your goal is being more attractive: There is a direct connection between exercise and healthy, gorgeous skin and hair. Regular physical activity will give you: (1) better collagen production, which leads to smoother, firmer skin, (2) reduced acne, and (3) healthier hair. You can get these benefits from all types of activity!

If your goal is living a longer life: According to a 2012 review of exercise studies (10), participants who got at least 150 minutes (2 hours and 30 minutes) of moderate activity a week were anticipated to up to 6 extra years compared to those who were less active. There are no rules for what activity you have to do to reap those benefits—just that you're moving during that time.

If your goal is getting in better aerobic/cardiovascular shape: Training to improve aerobic and cardiovascular performance should include work at all intensities. To be truly aerobically fit, dedicate training time to low-, moderate-, and high-intensity heart rate zones. An excellent method for achieving this is to include interval training in your workout where you will raise and lower the intensity, working at a high rate in short bursts.

If your goal is improving your numbers: Getting more physical activity can have a profound effect on your "numbers," like blood pressure, cholesterol, and waist size. All of these are indicators of heart health and overall wellness. Even better, changes in these numbers are measurable, concrete ways to track your efforts.

If your goal is preparing for an event: If you're training for an event, such as a race, fun run, marathon, or even dance marathon, get some support and motivation from others. See if there is a training program for your event, such as Team in Training, or an online group of people you can train with. Having that event date in mind is great motivation and can help you figure out a training schedule to get you to where you need to be by event day.

7. What motivates you to be healthier?

- Feeling myself get healthier and improving my well-being

- Being more attractive
- Having fun
- Being an example for others
- Having support from friends and/or family
- My doctor wants me to
- It's expected of me

If you are motivated by feeling yourself get healthier and improving your well-being: No matter what you are striving to be healthy for, increasing your physical activity arms your body against disease, strengthens your immune system, and increases your energy.

If you are motivated by being more attractive: All that work and sweat will pay off when it comes to beauty. To enhance the beautiful skin benefits that a regular work out gives you, make sure you are drinking enough water. An easy guideline for how much you should drink is (your weight in pounds)/2 = the number of ounces of water you should consume daily. On days that you work out, add another 16-24 ounces to that number.

If you are motivated by having fun: Being active isn't about torture. If you're having fun, you're far more likely to keep up with the activity and benefit from it. If you're taking a fun fitness class or have discovered your love for long power walks, enlist some friends to join you so you can share the enjoyment.

If you are motivated by being an example for others: Be a model for your friends and loved ones by showing them it's possible and fun to add physical activity to a daily routine. When you are at your best physically and mentally, you are the best help to others.

If you are motivated by having support from friends and/or family: Gather together some friends, a parent, a child —just about anybody—to foster fun and encouragement while getting active.

If you are motivated because your doctor wants you to be healthier: So your doctor says you need more physical activity. That's likely true of most women in America. Use your doctor as a partner and supporter in your exercise. Find out if there are specific suggestions he or she has that will maximize the benefits of being active.

If you are motivated because it's expected of you to be healthier: Exercise is a gift you give yourself for your health, longevity, wellness, and happiness. Even if you're expected by others in your life to be fit, ultimately, you're taking care of yourself and other people's opinions and expectations should take a smaller role in your life.

8. What keeps you from exercising or incorporating more activity into your schedule?

- **No time**
- **No motivation**
- **Too many commitments**
- **No energy**
- **Pain**
- **Housekeeping and chores**
- **Work/school hours**
- **The expense**
- **Not understanding how to achieve my movement goals**
- **No interest**
- **My kids**
- **No support from friends/family**
- **I'm embarrassed to have people see me exercising**

If you lack time: Each day, engage in at least one activity that gets your body moving. Even activities that don't seem like exercise—such as vacuuming, walking home from the train, or dancing at a club—can be beneficial.

If you lack motivation: Try rewarding yourself each time you exercise. This can be a material reward, or it can be something like 10 minutes of guilt-free social media scrolling. You can also motivate yourself by tracking your progress to see how you've improved.

If you have too many commitments: Try to make some of your family and social time active. Play outside with the kids, go on a walk or shopping trip with your friends, or even just park a little farther away when you're running your errands.

If you lack energy: Surprisingly, a brief, low- to moderate-intensity workout can pep you right up. Getting your blood flowing oxygenates your body, including your brain, and wakes you up. It also has a hormonal effect that boosts your energy, too.

If you have pain: Everything can seem like a challenge when you're in pain, but it doesn't have to stop you from living your life and being active however you can. Your doctor, physical therapist, or a personal trainer can help you find activities that give you all of the health benefits but none of the stress and pain of other types of exercise. Yoga, water aerobics, and the recumbent bike are just a few of the many exercise options for those in pain.

If you have housekeeping and chores: Make your chores and errands into a movement experience by picking up the pace in your cleaning with some lively music or by parking a little farther from the grocery store or dry cleaners. Housework and regular errands can be a great way to move around, and they count as activity.

If you are bound by work/school hours: Find some time in your work or study schedule to take breaks. Your body needs the opportunity to refresh and re-energize in order for you to be at your best mentally. Get up and walk or do a few stretches.

It is very important for you to schedule in times when you can devote 20 minutes or more to moderate exercise. Consider this a necessary step toward your success at work or school.

If you have trouble with the expense: Being active does not mean having a $100 per month gym membership—unless you want it to! There are many free and low-cost options that will have just as many benefits as a gym membership. Local universities and community centers often have free or low-cost fitness classes and access to gym equipment and pools. There's always YouTube for countless quality, free workout videos from great instructors. You can also go low-tech and walk your neighborhood or high school track. For strength training, your own body weight is all you need to shape up. Movements like push-ups, sit-ups, leg lifts, and the like sculpt beautiful muscles for free.

If you lack understanding of how to achieve your movement goals: The hardest part of exercise is setting goals, but all that work is for nothing if you don't know how to achieve those goals. Once you have your movement goals set, consult a personal trainer, a fitness instructor, or your doctor for ways to achieve those goals.

If you lack interest: "Physical activity" can happen outside of the gym and outside of your assumptions about what exactly it constitutes. What do you love to do that doesn't involve sitting in a chair? Boating? Shopping? Dancing? Any activity where you're moving is, by definition, physical activity. You may not break a sweat, but if you're in motion, you're on the right track.

If you are bound by kids: Children are built-in workout partners. Whether you're chasing them around the yard, cleaning up after them, or corralling them, you're in constant motion. Get into a child's mindset and think about opportunities to play.

If you lack support from friends/family: Online support

groups, message boards, and social networking sites provide a wide world of people just like you who want to talk and support each other.

If you are embarrassed to have people see you exercising: Everyone is too focused on themselves to watch you at the gym. Promise! However, there is plenty that can be done in the privacy of your own home. Run stairs, do a workout DVD, try a few YouTube exercise videos. Being active is only as public as you want it to be.

9. **If all of these barriers above were removed, could you achieve your goals?**

- Yes
- No

If yes: Okay! This is something we can work with. For each of the barriers you identified in question 8, think of how you could work around it or eliminate it completely. No need to ground yourself in reality right now. If it would take a personal chef to get you to eat well, write it down. You can find a more realistic solution later.

If no: In an ideal world, what would make you able to achieve what you want? Is this even something you do want? How can you find your way around anything else standing in your way?

Activity Guidelines

In addition to the dietary guidelines, the Centers for Disease Control and Prevention (3) publishes a physical activity guidelines report for adult Americans aged 18-64. This report provides aerobic and muscle-strengthening guidance for healthy adults and adults with special health statuses (e.g., pregnant or disabled) for physical activity beyond ordinary daily activities , like showering or tying your shoes. Aerobic activity is any physical activity that causes you to move large muscles (arms, torso, legs) in a rhythmic manner over a sustained period of time. This can be as simple as walking the dog for a half hour, dancing, taking a fitness class, swimming, jogging, or cleaning the house.

Muscle-strengthening activity is activity that makes your muscles do more work than they are accustomed to doing in daily life. Think of this as lifting items that are heavier than normal, including using your own body weight. You can be a traditionalist with dumbbells and weight machines, or you can do yoga, Pilates, or anything else that makes your muscles work.

The CDC (3) provides the following key guidelines for adults without special health status (we'll get to special health states next):

- Avoid being inactive. Some physical activity—even in small doses—is better than none. Any amount of activity can provide benefits in how you feel physically and mentally.
- To get the most health benefits from being active, adults should do at least 150 minutes (2 hours and 30 minutes) a week of moderate-intensity, or 75 minutes (1 hour and 15 minutes) a week of vigorous-intensity aerobic physical activity, or some combination of moderate- and vigorous-intensity aerobic activity. For those looking to reap the most benefits from activity, aerobic activity should be performed in bouts of at least ten minutes, and preferably, it should be spread throughout the week.

- For the overachievers, CDC recommends 300 minutes (five hours) a week of moderate-intensity, or 150 minutes a week of vigorous-intensity aerobic physical activity, or some combination throughout the week to get the most extensive health benefits.
- In addition to the aerobic activity recommendations, CDC recommends that adults do muscle-strengthening activities that are moderate or high intensity two days a week. These activities should cover all major muscle groups throughout the week —not necessarily all on one day. Unsurprisingly, including the muscle-strengthening activity will increase the benefits from exercise even more.

Bottom line: do more, and you'll get more out of it. We will discuss exactly what you'll get later in this pillar. For those who are feeling overwhelmed by these activity guidelines, don't worry. If you are not currently active, you'll be working gradually toward these activity levels. You'll make progress by spreading short periods of light-to-moderate intensity exercise throughout the week.

If you are currently active, you will likely maintain your current activity level, but vary the activity types and focus more on other chances for movement.

Guidelines for Postpartum Women

Women who are in the postpartum period are recommended to be moderately active. The amount and type of activity is a matter for your doctor, so be sure to speak to him or her before beginning a new exercise program.

The CDC (3) provides the following key guidelines for women during the postpartum period:

- Healthy women who are not already highly active or doing vigorous-intensity activity are recommended to get at least 150 minutes (2 hours and 30 minutes) of moderate-intensity aerobic activity each week during the postpartum period. Preferably, this activity should be spread throughout the week.

- If you are cleared by your doctor, women who already habitually engage in vigorous-intensity aerobic activity, or who are highly active, can continue physical activity during the postpartum period.

Guidelines for Adults with Disabilities and Chronic Medical Conditions

According to the CDC (3), the following guidelines are appropriate for adults with all types of disabilities and chronic medical conditions. Please discuss your activity with your doctor prior to beginning a new exercise program. In consultation with your doctor, you can determine the level of activity that is appropriate. If you are able to do moderate-to-high amounts of physical activity, you should follow the guidelines for healthy adults above. Otherwise, the CDC recommends the following:

- As you are able, you should do at least 150 minutes (2 hours and 30 minutes) a week of moderate-intensity, or 75 minutes (1 hour and 15 minutes) a week of vigorous-intensity aerobic physical activity, or some combination of moderate- and vigorous-intensity aerobic activity. For those looking to reap the most benefits, aerobic activity should be performed in bouts of at least ten minutes, and preferably, it should be spread throughout the week.

- As you are able, the CDC recommends including muscle-strengthening activities that are moderate or high intensity two days a week. These activities should cover all major muscle groups throughout the week—not necessarily all on one day.
- When you aren't able to meet these guidelines, you should be physically active regularly, according to your abilities, and avoid inactivity.

I can't stress this enough: speak with your doctor before making any activity changes. There are many ways to be active, and knowing what will work best for you is key.

About Movement

There are many ways to look at movement. Sure, there are the hard-core gym goers, yoga queens, and long distance runners out there. You might even be one of them. That level of fitness can be a lot of fun and can bring people lots of joy. But, there's a difference between fitness and activity. Most of us say we want to get in better shape. What does that mean to you? Are you talking about being stronger, more flexible, or having better endurance? If so, that's fitness.

Fitness has to do with your strength, vigor, athleticism, muscularity, and so on. There is such a thing as being overweight but fit. Fitness goals are great for people at any size or current fitness level. Maybe this isn't your first rodeo. Perhaps you've tried to exercise before and it just didn't work for you. That might be because when you say you want to get in better shape, you really mean you want to lose weight. In that case, we're talking about activity, because "weight loss" is code for "fat loss." The way to use up your fat stores is through low- to moderate-intensity activity, like casual swimming or brisk walking, rather than fitness work.

Fitness is achieved through a variety of low-, medium-, and high-intensity cardiovascular exercise, flexibility work, and strength training. Further, fitness is enhanced by agility, endurance, and explosiveness training. If that made your head spin, don't worry. I have a guide in this section that shows you the exact exercises you can do if fitness is your goal.

Activity is just moving. In other words, moving around more than you are sedentary. This includes low-intensity movement like walking, playing in the pool, yoga, getting in steps on your Fitbit, taking the stairs, and other easy things to fit into your life. Ideally, you'd have a combination of fitness and activity goals in your plan. That leads to overall health and works like gangbusters in conjunction with a nutritious diet to let you live your most energetic and amazing life. I'm going to work off the assumption that you will have fitness and activity goals, but you do you. If you're just trying to get in 5,000 steps a day, you're still in the right place.

There are many reasons why people struggle with exercise. One of the most common reasons is that they don't have a structured program that works for them. They might not even know where to start. Another reason is that they don't have realistic goals. It's easy to set huge goals and then just give up when they are more difficult to achieve than you thought . . . which they probably will be. Maybe in the past you've dreaded exercise because you just didn't choose a fitness program that made you feel excited or motivated. What works for others may be torture for you. Commit to choosing exercise that you like. There are endless possibilities for both activity-based movement and fitness-based exercises. Set realistic goals and choose exercises that make you smile. If you're not enjoying yourself, at least a little bit, then you're not as likely to follow through.

Often associated with fitness goals, cardiovascular exercise is exercise that gets your heart pumping. You breathe more heavily and your heart rate increases. Cardio helps you build endurance and strengthens your heart and lungs. It's an important part of any exercise program, whether you are trying to lose weight or reach fitness goals. Many people mistakenly believe that cardio has to be intense and that you need to be breathing heavily and really pushing yourself in order to get any benefit. This isn't true at all. In fact, cardio exercise is best thought of as a moderate- or low-intensity exercise. On an exertion scale of 1-10, you should be right in the middle, around a 5. That means when you're doing the exercise, you should be able to hold a conversation. You may feel a bit winded, but you should feel like you could continue at the same pace for quite a long time. For those looking to increase fitness or just curb boredom, try interval training. This involves alternating periods of low-, medium-, and bursts of high-intensity exercise. For example, walking on treadmill at a low intensity for one minute, cranking up the speed or incline slightly for a fast walk or light jog for 30 seconds, upping the speed or incline again to where you are sprinting for 15 seconds, then going all the way back down to low intensity. Then you keep repeating the cycle.

When people think about cardio exercise, running is often the first thing that comes to mind. And then they cringe, go back to bed, and forget this whole "exercise" thing. If you don't like running, then don't run. Yep, that's right. Just forget it. Think about something that gets your heart pumping just a little harder than normal. This might be something like riding your bike. Jumping rope, hula hooping, and swimming are all cardio, too. Some activities you might not immediately consider include sports like tennis or basketball and martial arts activities like karate. Think about an activity you enjoy or would like to learn how to do. For example, if you've always wanted to try kickboxing then now is the time. If you used to play tennis when you were younger and would love to play again, that may be your cardio focus. If you have beautiful trails in your area and enjoy nature, then maybe your cardio will be hiking. Identify an activity or two you can do and are interested in.

We all start at different fitness levels. Maybe you can't remember the last time you exercised and increased your heart rate. That's fine. Maybe you exercise once in a while, or you're a weekend warrior, and you simply want to make your fitness more regular. Your present fitness level isn't the focus. It's the starting point, and it's how you'll decide what steps to take next. Go out and spend 30 or 40 minutes doing your thing. For example, if you decided that you're going to do Zumba, then find an online Zumba class, borrow a DVD from the library, or head to a beginner class. Keep your heart rate at a moderate level so that you feel like you're working out, but you don't feel exhausted. Remember that you should be able to carry on a conversation while you exercise. Then evaluate:

- How'd it go?
- Do you feel good?
- Was that the right activity for you?
- Did you choose your intensity level well?

If you pushed yourself too hard (or maybe took it too easy), that's okay; it's a learning moment. Learning to pace yourself is a skill and not one that most people are very good at. If you disliked the activity itself, then repeat this test with a different activity. If you don't know what to do or where to start, then just put on your walking shoes and get outside. Walk at a brisk pace and enjoy the fresh air.

Here's the mistake most people make, why so many goals fail, and why people give up: they start too hard. They push their bodies too much. The workout they choose is too intense. It feels terrible and then they form opinions like "I hate running" or "exercise stinks." Pick something you'd like to do.

Here are some tips for exercise success:

- **Make it fun.** Music is a good way to add some fun and interest to the workout. You can also bring a friend or your dog. Go walk somewhere interesting. People watch. Join a gym with TVs.
- **Stagger the days where you work on fitness goals.** While I want you to be active every day, your heavy cardio and strength exercise shouldn't be daily. Your body needs time to rest and recover after a hard workout.
- **Create time.** I'm going to bet it's not easy to find time in your busy schedule. Create time. Get up earlier, change your lunch habits, eat dinner later. You're going to have to get creative here to find an extra 40 minutes in your day. But rest assured; it's worth it. You're going to begin feeling wonderful. Maybe you can multitask and call your mom while walking or listen to an audiobook.
- **Be patient.** This is going to be the hardest one. I bet you have a planner full of things to do and want to see progress from your effort, like, yesterday. Most of us like instant gratification. We can watch a movie or buy a sweater with the click of a button. Exercise doesn't work like that. You're not going to be able to notice much change in your body after just a week of exercise. You may not feel that exercise rush you're hoping for. For the first month it may feel like a struggle to make this a habit. Stick with it. You will begin to see changes. You will find that your workouts get easier and you need to make things more challenging. Hopefully, you will feel that surge of endorphins that will make you smile for hours afterward, and your exercise will become a natural habit.

If you have fitness-based goals, you must include strength training. This is where the real results are going to begin taking shape, literally, since your body shape will change. Like cardio, strength training is whatever you make of it. It can be lifting heavy weights in the gym or it can be bodyweight exercises in your living room. By definition, strength training is a type of exercise that uses resistance to induce muscular contraction. This movement builds the strength, anaerobic endurance, and size of skeletal muscles. Strength training uses a different energy system than cardiovascular exercise. Where cardio uses aerobic energy (with oxygen being part of the energy equation), strength training does not use oxygen. Anaerobic systems actually burn sugar, generally through a process known as glycolysis, for energy. This is another important piece of the puzzle in your overall fitness and health.

Many women avoid strength training because they believe it will make them bulky. Let's be extremely clear here. The only way a woman is going to get bulky from strength training is if she already has a significant layer of fat over the muscle or she is taking something. You're not going to get bulky. What you will get is more developed muscle tissue and a leaner body. Muscle burns more calories than fat, and as you replace fat with muscle, you'll boost your burn. You'll begin to see changes in your body. If you hope to drop a jean size or have other appearance-based goals, then adding strength training to your program is a must. On that note, let's take a look at strength training exercises you can do.

Just like cardio, it's important that you have a little fun with your training. Find exercises and programs you enjoy. I'm going to go through a few of the most common types of strength training.

First is body weight exercise. You'd be surprised how much simple bodyweight exercises can change your body shape and how difficult they can be. Don't believe it? Drop and do 100 pushups. Yep, a pushup is a bodyweight strength training exercise. Sit-ups are, too. And if you can do 100 bodyweight squats without your leg muscles burning, then you're in better shape than I am. Other bodyweight exercises include lunges, planks, pull-ups, or chin-ups.

Next are barbells and dumbbells. You can also invest in a home gym or head to a nearby recreation center or gym and use their weights. Keep in mind that when you start lifting weights, it's a good idea to have someone demonstrate proper form. If you're lifting heavy weights and you have improper form, you can get hurt.

Then we have kettlebells. Kettlebells are little cast-iron weights with a handle. They come in a wide variety of weights from 12 pounds to 70 pounds (or more). Essentially, you can use them like you'd use a dumbbell.

There are also resistance bands. Resistance bands are like long rubber bands. Generally, when you purchase resistance bands, they're purchased in a package with varying degrees of tension. The harder it is to stretch the band, the more resistance and the more difficult the movement.

Remember that test that you did for your cardio program? It's a good idea to do the same thing with strength training. You might consider starting with a bodyweight program first. This is particularly important if you've never done any type of strength training before. A bodyweight program will help you become aware of and familiar with the exercise movements and with your muscles. You can also do it anywhere with a little floor space and without needing equipment!

Keep in mind that you're going to be doing cardio several times a week as well. Now, it's time to add strength training to your plan. There are two approaches to consider. One approach is to combine strength training and cardio into one day. You can do 20 minutes of strength training after your cardio for a full hour workout. You can also do strength training on the "off days" from cardio. Ideally, you want to get to the point where you're strength training three to four times a week. Consider also performing mobility and flexibility work on your off days. You might do some gentle yoga at home or stretch and work on mobility. This will help reduce any muscle soreness.

I've made a guide of workout ideas that you can use to put together workouts of your choice. It includes both strength and cardio movements that are almost all equipment-free! Download it for free from my website (see the QR code in the Introduction).

Making Workouts Harder

If you've been working out for a while now, but you want to progress further to reach your goals, here are some ways you can make your workouts harder so you can keep challenging yourself.

- Use more weight or resistance—carefully and slowly add weight or resistance and see how you feel
- Add more reps or time—but don't do this at the same time as adding weight
- Use free weights or kettlebells instead of machines—this will challenge you in a new way without changing weight or reps
- Change your stability—do your set on one leg, a Bosu ball, or other surface that requires you to work on balancing while you move
- Try circuit training—keep moving through your circuit to keep your heart rate up
- Increase your range of motion—twist, squat, bend, or reach farther
- Add an incline on the treadmill—no need to change your speed!

- Add intervals—alternate periods of high-intensity and low-intensity exercise

Now that we've tackled the movement side of your program, we're ready to move on to its all-important counterpart, nutrition.

PILLAR FIVE: NUTRITION

Nutrition

Balance is important in your diet for weight loss, energy, and overall health. If you'll take yourself back to elementary school, there are certain groups of food our bodies need—fruits and vegetables, protein, and grains. We have so many options for getting the produce, protein, and grains we need these days that having a balanced, healthy diet is possible on any budget with any dietary challenges. Your goal is to feed yourself the fuel you need for optimal performance, which means vitamin-rich, fiber-filled, whole foods. I have some suggestions for the budget-conscious folks at the end of this chapter, so don't fret if you think you need to be a regular at Whole Foods or organic juice bar to be healthy.

Media, athletes, and that guy at work all talk a lot about protein—maybe too much. Protein is important, that's true. However, unless you're a bodybuilder or only exist on food from the vending machine, you're probably getting enough protein already. Yep, you too, vegetarians. Protein is found in more than just meat and powders. Fruit, vegetables, legumes, nuts, seeds, dairy, eggs, and grains also have protein in them. Tracking your protein intake for a week or two will give you an idea of where you stand. It's recommended that women consume a minimum of .36 grams of protein per pound of body weight per day. So, if you weigh 130 pounds, that means you should shoot for at least 47 grams of protein daily. This changes if you are pregnant, nursing, under a lot of stress, or engaging in either endurance or strength training. If you are pregnant, nursing, or under unusual stress, please speak with your doctor about your dietary needs. For the athletes, there are many good protein calculators you can find online if you are doing strength or endurance training.

As a general rule, you can use the following calculations for daily protein needs:

- Endurance training requires .55 to .64 grams of protein per pound of body weight per day.
- Strength training requires .73 to .78 grams of protein per pound of bodyweight per day.
- Endurance and strength training together are also .73 to .78 grams of protein per pound of bodyweight per day.
- Pregnant women generally need an extra 10 grams of protein per day above suggested levels. Talk to your OB, though.
- Nursing women typically need 15 grams per day extra the first 6 months and 12 grams per day extra the second six months. You should talk to your OB about this, too.

Don't attempt to be an overachiever and eat as much protein as possible. Eating more than 35 percent of your total daily calories in protein is too much. Excess protein can't be stored in the body, so eating too much may put a strain on your kidneys and liver.

If you are upping your exercise significantly to reach your goals, or you feel a little sluggish after working out, think about your protein timing. When you're strength training, it's important to get some protein into your body within 30 minutes after you've finished your workout. This will help reduce muscle soreness and improve your recovery time so you can stay on your exercise schedule. As you continue with your strength training and start moving into heavier movements and weights, protein may become more important. Regarding that post-workout protein intake, don't make this difficult. You could have a protein shake or smoothie, but that can be a pain. You'd do just as well with a glass of milk, string cheese, hard-boiled egg, low-sugar protein bar, or some nuts.

Even if you didn't live through the low-fat craze of the 90s, you likely have heard of the Atkins, South Beach, and low-carb frenzy of the early 2000s and the modern versions of it today. Carbs are the fuel that your body turns to for energy. There are many myths about carbs, but the most prevalent is the belief that all carbs are bad. Carbohydrates are not bad guys. For example, a carrot is a carbohydrate. So is a cupcake. You can probably guess which source of carbs is better for you. When it comes to the carbs you should limit, try to avoid anything that has refined flour or added sugar. That's what we'd call junk food. I'm not immune to a slice of cake or a bread basket, and you don't need to swear off of these types of carbs. Just use them sparingly when planning your diet. You'll have more energy. Your body will turn to your fat stores for energy instead of your sugar stores during workouts. You'll lose fat faster and also reduce your risk for cancer, diabetes, and cardiovascular disease.

While you're limiting your intake of junky carbs, boost your intake of the good ones. This includes vegetables, fruit, and whole grains. One method I have found works well is to crowd out the bad with the good. The more quality carbs you're eating, the more satisfying fiber you're getting. This takes care of hunger and doesn't leave room to fill up on junk that will only temporarily fix your craving.

Your diet is hugely important to your success, but please don't try to make big changes right now. Small changes that are manageable are a smarter path to success. For example, instead of trying to eliminate sugar or stop eating all junk food, you might cut back on sugar or limit your junk food to just twice a week. Trust that as you begin to take better care of your body through small, incremental dietary changes, your goals will come. This brings us to some simple lifestyle changes you can begin making. Keep in mind that a proper diet and exercise go hand-in-hand. The better you eat, the faster you'll lose weight, the more energy you'll have, and the more successful your workouts will be. As you notice changes in your body, energy level, and mindset, you'll feel motivated to push forward toward your goals.

Like I said, going all-in on dietary changes is tempting, but you'll burn out quickly and feel deprived. Here are four changes you can start with that will make a big dent in your goals.

Eat breakfast. There are many things you can do to make breakfast fast and easy. Make a breakfast smoothie. Enjoy a cup of Greek yogurt with fruit. Make egg muffins in advance and pop them in the microwave for a quick reheat. Breakfast is important because it gives you the energy you need to stay fueled all day. The calories you take in from adding breakfast if you're normally a non-breakfast-eater will be more than made up for in your reduced need to snack or overeat later in the day.

Eat vegetables at every meal. Fiber is a wonderful thing. You'll find that the fiber in vegetables fills you up for only a few calories. In addition to weight loss effects, the vitamins in your vegetables will increase your overall health. You might even find that your skin, hair, and nails look better! Shift the focus on your plate at mealtime. Make vegetables the star and protein the side dish. Don't limit yourself to salads or sad steamed vegetables, either. There are tons of fantastic vegetable recipes to try.

Watch your calorie intake, but don't obsess over it. There's a terrible phenomenon where people gain weight when they start exercising. This happens for two reasons. First, they think they've burned off more calories than they actually have, and they reward themselves with a big meal or a treat food. Second, and more innocently, they finish a workout and find that they're very hungry so they consume a large meal or snack to regain energy. The result is the same as those who reward themselves. They eat more than they just burned off. Eat nutritiously before your workouts and consume a small protein-heavy snack afterward. Remember, exercising isn't an excuse to eat more or to replenish your electrolytes with beer, as my husband claims.

Finally, hydrate. Make sure you drink enough water throughout the day. Pace yourself, too. Chugging isn't as helpful as drinking consistently over the day. When you're dehydrated, it affects how your body moves nutrients and waste through itself. Dehydration also impacts how quickly your cells can make energy. A sign of dehydration is fatigue, and none of us can afford to be tired.

Now, if you're on a budget or are a savvy shopper, consider buying frozen fruit and vegetables. They are just as good for you as fresh, cost a fraction of the price, and they last longer. If you love fresh produce, consider getting a membership to Costco or a similar club. They have beautiful fresh fruit, vegetables, meats, cheeses, and anything else you can imagine. You can buy canned goods, too. I always have all sorts of beans, diced and crushed tomatoes, cans and boxes of broth, and corn.

They are cheap and long-lasting, and they are perfect to have on hand to make soup. Many others in this field recommend buying dry beans, which are cheap for sure, but I don't have time to deal with soaking and cooking them longer. But, if you love to cook or are on a budget, go for it. You can get incredible deals in the international foods section of your grocery store on dry beans and bags of rice. Lastly, Amazon Fresh and Amazon Pantry are also great low-cost ways to get your food. The biggest benefit is that you don't have to spend time shopping. They are also a bit cheaper than the grocery store delivery services like Peapod and Instacart.

Nutrition Guidelines

Food is not our enemy. You do not need to go to battle with it. Food is energy to keep your body moving so you can do what you love to do. That said, though food's primary purpose is nourishment, it is also something for you to enjoy. Eating healthfully and enjoying food aren't mutually exclusive. To get the most out of your nutrition, the U.S. Department of Agriculture (USDA) (13) publishes dietary guidelines to help Americans eat a healthier diet. The USDA recommends a diet that includes:

- A variety of vegetables from all of the different subgroups: dark green, red, orange, starchy, beans, and peas
- Fresh, whole fruits (rather than canned or fruit juices)
- Grains, where at least half of your intake is from whole grains
- Fat-free or low-fat dairy from sources like milk, yogurt, and cheese

- Proteins, including seafood, lean meats, poultry, eggs, legumes, nuts, seeds, and soy
- Healthy fats and oils

The guidelines also recommend that a healthy diet limits:

- Trans fats and keeps saturated fat to less than 10 percent of calories per day
- Added sugars, so that less than 10 percent of calories per day are from added sugars
- Added sodium, not to exceed 2,300 mg per day
- Alcohol to one drink per day for women

I have free regular and vegetarian 14-day meal plans that can be used as-is or as guides for you to create your own plan that matches your tastes. Download them for free from my website (see the QR code in the Introduction).

Sensory Hunger

The food industry, chefs, culinary magazines—they have all mastered the art of palatability or the perception of tastiness. Palatability is mostly based on how the food stimulates our senses, including memories of when we had good or bad experiences with the food. Usually, the foods we find most appealing are visually appealing and smell good. The trick with the palatability of food is the senses it has engaged. Have you ever been full after a meal, so completely full that you couldn't dare to eat another bite? What happened when dessert came out? Did you find a way to eat another bite since it looked so good?

How about when you haven't even thought about food. You're out and about, busy and not ready for a meal. Have you ever experienced the smell of something you love, like popcorn at a movie theater or pizza? Suddenly, you could eat. Your senses are stimulating your appetite. It's this sensory stimulation (or the thought of that stimulation) instead of actual hunger that drives us to eat when we aren't hungry. When we habitually seek out that sensory stimulation as the primary driver for eating instead of eating for hunger and enjoying the sensory aspect as a bonus, we end up overeating.

Mindful Eating

Eating mindfully is all about taking it slow and enjoying your food for what it is. Learning how to eat mindfully is one of the most effective tools for a positive connection with food. With such busy lifestyles and so many distractions, many of us are guilty of "inhaling" our food without much pleasure, just so we can fill up quickly and move onto our next task. Maybe you eat in the car or over the sink? Perhaps you barely remember choosing what to eat and eating it.

When you eat faster than your body can cope with, you end up eating more than your body really needs, resulting in overeating without realizing it. From the time you start eating, it takes around 20 minutes for your brain to send signals to your body that you are full. Slower, more mindful eating allows your body enough time to trigger the signal from your brain that you've had enough. It also gives you the simple pleasure of enjoying your food. Without that, you might as well just consume nutrient-rich gruel!

So, how do you eat mindfully? Start with taking it slow. Each and every time you are about to eat (even if it's just a handful of nuts), the first thing you should do is pause for a moment, have a quick think about the food and if your body needs it. By looking at what you are about to eat, you are able to see if it's something you really need or just want. Simply wanting food is fine, so long as you slow down to enjoy it.

Before you eat, take a moment to use your senses. Take deep breaths to enjoy the smell of the food. Be aware of how the food looks, including the plate, table, and anything around you. What do you hear? Is it quiet? Do you hear music and conversation? Taking time to use your senses heightens your awareness for what you are eating and allows your body time to enjoy the process. Culturally, our appreciation of the eating experience can be limited simply to the energy the food gives us. If you're with others, take in the pleasure of their company. If you're alone, focus on how nice it is to have a moment of peace.

Between mouthfuls, take nice deep breaths so your body can have time to digest the food and so that you have time to enjoy it. Put your feet firmly on the ground and sit upright with your cutlery on the table while you chew. By giving your body the space to do its job in between bites, you become aware of when you are full and how you feel when you eat certain foods.

Think of it like this: When you are in a hurry, you drive, right? When you want to take it slow you walk or ride your bike or take the bus. Well, just remember to take the BUS next time you sit down to eat:

- B – Breathe
- U – Use your senses
- S – Slow down

Taming Your Eating Triggers

If you're like lots of busy, overachieving women, you occasionally fall victim to stress eating or "emotional eating." This is when you use food to comfort yourself or mask your feelings and emotions.

When it comes to emotional eating there is always a trigger point. That trigger is what kicks off behavior, and it's usually caused by an emotion or reaction to a situation. For example, seeing cookies in the breakroom at work may be a trigger for eating junk you don't want. Another trigger may be working late which causes you to be too tired to find nutritious food. Once you know your trigger point, it's easy to see the action you take afterwards that leads you to eat emotionally.

The first step to keeping your triggers from leading you down an emotional eating path is to figure out the feeling you have when you start emotionally eating. This is the time to be brutally open and honest with yourself. Be objective. The better you can analyze your triggers and responses, the more effective your plan to tame them will be.

This is a list of the most common triggers that can lead to emotional eating:

- Anger
- Anxiousness
- Boredom
- Depression
- Disappointment
- Disconnection
- Envy
- Fear
- Frustration
- Greed
- Insecurity
- Jealousy
- Laziness
- Loneliness
- Sadness
- Shame
- Stress

Over the next few days, pay attention to how you react to stressful situations and when you experience feelings like I listed above. For example, "I'm bored because my friend canceled last-minute, and now I'm home alone," or "I'm angry because I worked hard on that project and wasn't recognized for it." Think about some of those triggers, and then turn the reaction around from eating your feelings to doing something more constructive.

Think about why you react a certain way to your triggers. If you can get an idea of your "whys" for recent emotional eating episodes, you can analyze potential actions for dealing with them. Oftentimes, we resort to food to fill in that void and turn the negative emotion into a positive one. By doing this, we aren't allowing ourselves time to process and cope with the emotion. Remember that emotional eating isn't always a result of negative emotions. You can eat out of happiness at a party or closeness at a family event.

Here are some examples of triggers and the reactions you might have when eating emotionally:

Trigger: You are feeling stressed out because you have to reach a deadline at work and you might not make it.

Reaction: You go to the office vending machine and grab a chocolate bar or bag of chips to calm your nerves.

Trigger: You are angry because you had an argument with your spouse this morning and it has made your day feel like it will be long and terrible.

Reaction: You grab a caramel latte and a muffin on the way to work to suppress the anger and counteract the anticipation of a bad day.

Trigger: You are upset because your friend hurt your feelings and you feel betrayed.

Reaction: You go home and sit on the couch with a tub of ice cream to feel better.

Trigger: You feel lonely because your partner has been

traveling for work constantly and you need to raise the kids solo.

Reaction: You snack on cookies and candy throughout the day to cope and feel better.

Trigger: You won an award for community service and you're riding high.

Reaction: You overindulge on celebratory drinks with friends to commemorate the win.

All triggers can be managed in a way that prevents you from reaching for food as a way to cope instead of directly addressing your feelings. Right now, your habit might be to turn to food when emotions or stress arise. So, instead of trying to break the habit, we could try to simply replace the bad reaction with a good reaction. It will be the same trigger but a different reaction, making it much easier to change. Remember, baby steps.

Let's change the reactions from the triggers listed above by replacing them with a "good" reaction that is more beneficial:

Trigger: You are feeling stressed out because you have to reach a deadline at work and you might not make it.

New Reaction: You go for a five minute walk outside to get some fresh air to calm your nerves.

Trigger: You are angry because you had an argument with your spouse this morning and it has made your day feel like it will be long and terrible.

New Reaction: You take five minutes to write down your emotions and feelings to clear your head and handle the situation better.

Trigger: You are upset because your friend hurt your feelings and you feel betrayed.

New Reaction: You do some jumping jacks and stretches to release the tension.

Trigger: You feel lonely because your partner has been

traveling for work constantly and you need to raise the kids solo.

New Reaction: You call a friend and check in to see how they are doing.

Trigger: You won an award for community service and you're riding high.

New Reaction: You plan a movie night or spa visit with your friends to celebrate.

If at any time you aren't sure what action to take in place of turning to food, just get up and go for a five minute walk to get some air and think about something completely different. If you can't do that, hit up YouTube for some funny videos.

Pick one trigger you want to focus on. This worksheet is also in the free program workbook on my website at www.tsirona.com/ybbbook (see the QR code in the Introduction).

- What is your trigger?
- Why does this tend to happen?
- What do you normally do/eat when this happens?
- What positive action can you replace the reaction with?
- How long do you think you'll need to focus on changing your reaction to make it a healthier habit? (One week, two weeks, one month?)

The best way to overcome a trigger is to set reminders in your calendar or on your phone at times when you are most likely to experience it. Here is an example: An afternoon lull hits you at around 3 p.m. each day at the office, even if you are busy, so you turn to the cookie jar and a can of soda. You might switch this action with going into the courtyard and doing some deep breathing or just sitting quietly for 10 minutes. With this example, you would set reminders in your phone for 2:45 p.m. to "Go to the courtyard for your afternoon breather," then again at 3 p.m. and again at 3:15 p.m. to help push you toward the positive action.

Once you feel like you don't need the reminder, you can then start to work on another trigger in your life. Perhaps you might start with stress, and then, next month, you might move on to frustration. Just take your time and know that the process can take a few days or a few months.

A Note on Food Rules and the "Health Halo"

Hopefully this pillar has shown you that your nutrition doesn't have to be complicated. Unfortunately, well-meaning people out there—friends and family, health industry professionals, writers for women's magazines, producers for talk shows, and more—make this all sound hard. You do not need to be a vegan, go gluten-free, follow a Paleo diet, only eat organic foods, or follow other rules, unless those ways of eating appeal to you. There don't need to be rules if they make your life miserable. They just end up making everything seem so hard that we give up.

To make all of this more frustrating, there is a phenomenon called the "health halo." This happens when we overestimate the healthiness of food based on a single claim, like low-carb, low-fat, gluten-free, all-natural, or organic. Our brains use those keywords as a mental shortcut to make us equate those claims to a food being low-calorie or even nutritious.

I'd like you to primarily focus on eating real food when you are hungry, like fruit, vegetables, whole grains, dairy, meat, nuts—you know, the things that even a kid knows are healthy. Yes, that leaves room for treats, the occasional snack machine trip, and anything else in your food life that brings you joy. Break free from the effect of the health halo and the rules people arbitrarily place on food.

CHECK-IN

Well, check you out. You've made it through a few parts of your plan, and you're probably feeling good about your work. This midpoint in your plan is a time for reflection. When you were setting your goals, we discussed the importance of reflection—especially in light of self-awareness, mindfulness, and your attention to the program.

This is the point where I strongly suggest that you evaluate all you have done so far. What have you accomplished? What didn't work? What goals were just right? What goals need tweaks or complete scrapping? This is your plan, and there is no obligation to keep working toward goals that aren't right for you. Changing any behavior is about setting goals, working on them, reflecting, and adjusting. You're an ever-changing person with a dynamic life, so your goals need to be in line with your reality.

You're probably starting to reach some of your short-term goals. This is cause for celebration! Once you finish your celebration, it's time to get locked back into your plan. Depending on which goals you've accomplished, you may need to adjust or set new goals. I caution you not to change your level of effort. Simply change what that effort is going into.

Here are some ways to adjust your goals and overall plan at this midpoint:

- **Evaluate your tracking methods:** Is the information you're tracking telling you enough about your progress? There are many ways to track progress, so make sure you're using the one that shows you the data you need to effectively evaluate your efforts.
- **Learn more:** You have a good knowledge base right now just from reading up to this point, but maybe you'd like more information on a particular area, like eating to manage diabetes or learning how to powerlift. Branch out a bit and open yourself up even more to the wide world of movement, nutrition, and a healthy lifestyle.
- **Keep wins as wins:** You may be tempted to slack a little since you've done so well. Or, maybe you feel like you deserve a break. This is destructive thinking. Change things up, but don't lose the wins you've already chalked up. Don't let your old habits creep back in. They are old news. Focus instead on learning something new and keeping your lifestyle fresh and interesting to avoid the backslide.

Take time to write down what your goals were and your evaluation of them. This worksheet is also in the free program workbook on my website at www.tsirona.com/ybbbook (see the QR code in the Introduction).

1. Restate your goals and methods for tracking each of them.

2. Review the tracking data you've collected to assess where you have made progress, times when you did especially well, and times when you experienced challenges.
3. Compare your midpoint goal progress with your starting point. Can any of your goals be checked off as accomplished? Which ones will you continue on with? Which ones should be cut or replaced?
4. Where do you project you will be in your progress in six weeks? Six months? One year?
5. What do these results mean to you? What have you been able to do in your life as a result of your progress?
6. Have you been successful in your efforts so far? Why or why not?
7. Will it be necessary for you to modify your strategies for change in order to change behavior and improve your wellness area by the end of the second half?
8. What factors helped you to be successful (e.g., gym partner, meal planning service, spouse's support)?

PILLAR SIX: STRESS MANAGEMENT

All about Stress

Many women have no idea that their high-octane, busy lives are sabotaging their health. There is good stress (what drives us to succeed) and bad stress (like worry or being upset). Bad stress can have both major and minor health effects, and it shows up in mental, physical, and social ways.

Symptoms of stress include:

- Feeling tense
- Depression
- Poor memory
- Poor concentration
- Increased alcohol consumption
- Anger/hostility
- Difficulty making decisions
- Frequent mood swings
- Negative thinking
- Distractibility

- Excess smoking or eating
- Feeling overwhelmed or helpless

Chronic stress without relief increases the risk for a variety of major and minor health issues as well as safety issues, like an increase in accidents. Stress is something to take seriously because it might be normal to have it, but it's certainly not healthy or serving you well.

Health risks from prolonged stress include:

- Accidents
- Headaches
- Bowel disorders
- Poor digestion
- Skin disorders
- Eating disorders
- Emotional disorders
- Asthma attacks
- High blood pressure/strokes
- Colds/infections
- Backache
- Arthritis/immune disorders
- Heart attacks
- Cancer
- Ulcers
- Sexual dysfunction

Stress is driven by an imbalance in our lives. It is a nonspecific response of the body to any demand, and it can show up in many ways. Stress might be acute and time-limited or longer-term like a sequence of stressful events. But stress can also be a good thing. For example, good stress comes from stretching yourself, like in this program or at a new job, with a new baby, or planning a wedding. We're more familiar with bad stress, though. This kind of stress comes from bad relationships, over work, illness, and other negative life events.

Stressors are positive or negative things that upset or excite you. They are the causes of stress at onset and what keeps that stress going. Some examples are worry, emotional and physical pain, exercise, training for a race, planning for a new baby, and, of course, trying to do it all and be a superwoman. We do want some good stressors in life to keep us growing and moving, but bad stressors can end up impacting us fiercely.

When we have too much negative stress over time, it can have some major effects on our physical systems. Your body goes into survival mode, which increases your susceptibility to illness and slows your digestive system. This can lead to stress-related stomach aches, which certainly don't make you feel happier and better, so the stress continues. Prolonged negative stress also alters your endocrine system which regulates metabolism, growth and development, tissue function, sexual function, reproduction, sleep, and mood. Those are all critical functions for a healthy body and life. One hormonal effect of stress you may have heard of is the overproduction of the hormone cortisol. Cortisol, in healthy amounts, helps to control blood sugar levels, regulate metabolism, reduce inflammation, and assist with memory formulation. It also affects salt and water balance and helps control blood pressure. We want you to produce cortisol through good stressors, like exercise—not through stress

Too much cortisol slows the body's ability to remove triglycerides from the bloodstream. It also creates excessive central obesity, otherwise known as belly fat. Your waist circumference is related to your risk for heart disease and diabetes, so getting a cortisol belly is more than just an appearance issue. Tension and anxiety, as well as depression, are frequent emotional consequences of stress. These can cause cortisol to be released and overproduced, so it's important not just to manage stress, but also to be on top of your mental health and seek help when you sense abnormal emotions and patterns.

Men and women react to and cope with stress in different ways. While men feel less stress, this doesn't mean they don't experience as many stressors. Theirs is just a different way of experiencing and handling those stressors. Men tend to deal with stress through aggression and a fight-or-flight response. You may notice that men punch a wall, yell, or go for a drive when over-stressed. Women tend to feel stress more strongly and deeply. We have a variety of responses to stress, such as emotion (like crying) or impulsive action (like binge eating). Interestingly, women frequently "tend and befriend" their stress. During stress, women will care for their children, families, and loved ones (tend) and find support from their female friends (befriend). We're hardwired to have these responses, as women's bodies make chemicals that are believed to promote them, such as oxytocin, which has a calming effect, and estrogen, which boosts oxytocin's effects. As we age, our hormonal balance changes, and we become more susceptible to chronic stress and depression.

Holmes and Rahe Scale of Life Events

According to the Holmes and Rahe Scale of Life Events (6), some of the biggest stressors are both the good and bad kinds. You can see here that wonderful things, like pregnancy and retirement, are on the same list as the death of a spouse, though they're lower on the list. In general, our major stressors come from our jobs, illness or disability, money, and our social world.

The scale lists 43 stressful life events. Each event is assigned a different weight for stress. The higher the score, and the larger the weight of each event, the more likely one will become ill from stress. You can use this scale to calculate your stress to see what needs to be changed and how urgent it is for your health.

To score your stress levels, add up the weights for each event that has happened to you in the last two years and determine your score.

- Death of spouse (100)
- Divorce (73)
- Marital separation (65)
- Jail term (63)
- Death of close family member (63)
- Personal injury or illness (53)
- Marriage (50)
- Fired at work (47)
- Marital reconciliation (45)
- Retirement (45)
- Change in health of family member (44)
- Pregnancy (40)
- Sex difficulties (39)
- Gain of new family member (39)
- Business readjustment (39)
- Change in financial state (38)
- Death of close friend (37)
- Change to a different line of work (36)
- Change in number of arguments with spouse (35)
- A large mortgage or loan (31)
- Foreclosure of mortgage or loan (30)
- Change in responsibilities at work (29)
- Son or daughter leaving home (29)
- Trouble with in-laws (29)
- Outstanding personal achievement (28)
- Spouse begins or stops work (26)
- Begin or end school/college (26)
- Change in living conditions (25)

- Revision of personal habits (24)
- Trouble with boss (23)
- Change in work hours or conditions (20)
- Change in residence (20)
- Change in school/college (20)
- Change in recreation (19)
- Change in church activities (19)
- Change in social activities (18)
- A moderate loan or mortgage (17)
- Change in sleeping habits (16)
- Change in number of family get-togethers (15)
- Change in eating habits (15)
- Vacation (13)
- Christmas (12)
- Minor violations of the law (11)

Results

- 11-150—You have only a low to moderate chance of becoming ill in the near future.
- 150-299—You have a moderate to high chance of becoming ill in the near future.
- 300-600—You have a high or very high risk of becoming ill in the near future.

Preventing Stress

Some ways to prevent stress are:

- Planning ahead and managing your time better. This may take effort up front, but it will save you hassle and stress.
- Eliminating the unnecessary parts of your life, including obligations, social events, leadership

positions, family events, and even household clutter. Finding the unnecessary can be hard. For stay-at-home moms, I recommend thinking about how the house would run if you went back to work full time and had to figure it all out. Often, they find that kids can do more chores, they can outsource chores like cleaning and grocery delivery, and that they eliminate the unnecessary tasks that have taken over their lives at home. For the rest of my clients, I invite them to do a similar simplification exercise. Think about what you'd need to do to make everything continue to work in your life if you suddenly got the chance to travel or you weren't able to pack your schedule as much. Bottom line: simplify.

While simplifying, seek out the good, fun, and pleasant, and fill your life with activities that bring you joy. Sure, you have to go to work and you have to call your mom occasionally, but what about the other things you've jammed into your schedule?

Along with filling your life with the joyful, find an outlet for stress, like pleasurable social activities, exercise, hobbies, journaling, or having a long lunch with a friend you can talk to.

Do what's a little scary and be hyper-protective of your work-life balance. There are times in our lives when we have to hustle a little harder and work some longer hours, but that shouldn't be the norm. Consider the payoff for your long hours. Also, consider how you can be more efficient during working hours so you don't need to be burning the midnight oil so much.

Finally, know your personal signs of stress and catch it early before it is out of control. Observe how you react to stressful situations. Do you overeat? Get temperamental? Find your shoulders stuck up by your ears? Grit your teeth? Know your warning signs.

Make a prioritized list that covers work, lifestyle, and responsibilities. Put what *must* be done at the top and see what's left. Do you have some space in your schedule? Don't immediately fill it! Allow yourself some breathing room for relaxation and wiggle room for the unexpected.

What is on your dread list—the list of the things you hate doing. For example, I hate taking the trash out. I also hate making phone calls to places like the insurance company and the doctor's office. Your dread list can be anything from work, home, or elsewhere. What from that list can you outsource or get rid of? It may not be possible for everything, but I bet you can make a deal with your husband or roommate to trade dreaded chores.

Make sure that you build down-time into your schedule. Make time for fun, your hobbies, and naps. That down-time can be open completely and allow you to simply sit around. To create more down-time, focus and work smarter not harder for all parts of your life. You can group like activities and close errands or dedicate a power hour to certain activities.

Engage in only *necessary* relationships and activities. Necessary can also mean necessary for your sanity and happiness, you know. Get rid of emotional vampires and other terrible people, and don't waste any time feeling guilty about it. Be sure you choose the social, community, and volunteer obligations that are most fulfilling and learn to say "no" to the rest. This is your time and no one else is entitled to it.

Priority List: Make a prioritized list that covers work, lifestyle, and responsibilities. Put what *must* be done at the top and see what's left. Where can you find some breathing room? This worksheet is also in the free program workbook on my website at www.tsirona.com/ybbbook (see the QR code in the Introduction).

Dread List: A dread list is all of the things you hate doing. Your dread list can be anything from work, home, or elsewhere. What from this list can you outsource or get rid of? This worksheet is also in the free program workbook on my website at www.tsirona.com/ybbbook (see the QR code in the Introduction).

Emotional Intelligence

Before you can effectively manage your stress, we need to talk about emotions. There's a concept of emotional intelligence. The gist of it is that we all have varying degrees of awareness of, control over, and expression of our emotions. Our ability to manage emotions enables us to handle our relationships well. But, even if we're out of practice when it comes to emotional intelligence, it's something we can improve.

There are four areas of emotional intelligence that can make your relationships more or less stressful, depending on your skill level. The first is **self-awareness**. This is your ability to know your strengths and weaknesses, what you're feeling, and why you might be feeling that way. Self-awareness is the critical trait needed for you to make any changes in your life. This means you're able to assess your situation (any situation) and then know your own abilities well enough to figure out how to change.

The second area of emotional intelligence is **self-management**. This is all about being able to take action on what you know from your self-awareness. You use self-management to set goals and keep moving forward on them, even when there are time constraints, barriers, and all manners of happenings distracting you from accomplishing them.

Next, we have **empathy**. This is your ability to sense, read, and decipher how others feel.

This part of emotional intelligence will be most important when you are dealing with others in your life.

Finally, there are **skillful relationships**. This area focuses on your proficiency in forming and maintaining relationships. Having a support system of family, friends, health and fitness providers, and even friends online will increase your chances of success, so this area can directly impact your likelihood of staying on track with your plan.

While self-awareness and self-management are key to you forming and staying on a plan, your empathy and relationship skills will make the process easier.

Your emotional intelligence can grow as you learn more about yourself and how to interact with the world. The practice of mindfulness has risen in popularity because it helps you focus inward and build your self-awareness. Mindfulness is being aware of what leads to certain behaviors (like, when I'm tired, I'm more likely to order delivery food), and then being aware as the whole process plays out. This awareness empowers you to pinpoint a behavior you want to change and then either manage your environment to avoid the triggers or use your self-management skills to work toward a more positive outcome.

For example, let's say you have a fight with your best friend. You feel sad and a bit tired from the fight, so you figure you'll make yourself feel better with some ice cream. Before you know it, half of the tub is gone, and you don't feel any better.

Now, let's consider the same scenario, but with mindfulness used instead. You have a fight with your best friend, and you're feeling sad and tired. You know that your go-to when sad is to eat something sweet and watch TV. You also know that every time you've done this, you've eaten more than you intended and you've felt worse. You now decide to think of what you can do to take your mind off of the fight. You could throw in a load of laundry, walk the dog, or even just watch TV without the ice cream. Mindfulness helps you stop, think, assess, and choose the path you really want instead of working on auto-pilot.

To put things simply, mindfulness is about being curious rather than forcing yourself to do something or to think in a certain way. Curiosity lets you not only be aware of something in your life, but it also allows you to explore alternative outcomes than just your default reaction.

To make a big change to the way you do things, you need to be extremely curious about what it feels like when you eat a certain unhealthy food or do another unhealthy behavior.

Notice, but don't judge yourself here. By being curiously aware, you begin to notice the unhealthy behavior you are engaging in might not fulfill the need you had hoped it would. This awareness changes in your mind to a knowing. Through the evidence you gathered in your curious exploration, you are able to make an informed and unemotional determination. You've now used mindfulness to see what happens when you enact certain behaviors. You've learned how to get deep into your thoughts and actions like never before.

Use Your Brain for Stress Management

Mindfulness is used in many practices, but the HALT acronym comes to us from Alcoholics Anonymous as a way to stop (halt) and consider four physical or emotional conditions, that, if not taken care of, can lead you to act out behaviors that are not in line with your healthy lifestyle.

HALT stands for Hunger, Anger (or agitation), Loneliness, and Tiredness. In our case, we use HALT as a tool to increase self-awareness and engage your self-management skills. Think of it as a distinct action plan for your curious exploration of your actions and thoughts when you're feeling crappy. The next time you are about to lash out, get overwhelmed, give in to a craving, skip your daily physical activity, or do anything else that is detrimental, stop for a moment. Analyze whether you are about to perform the behavior because you are hungry, angry or agitated, lonely, or tired.

Let's talk about **hunger** first. This one is pretty self-explanatory. Have you eaten a nutritious meal or snack recently? Are you actually hungry, or do you just want a sleeve of cookies? My mom used to say, "If you're actually hungry, you'd be fine with an apple. If the apple won't work for you, you're not really hungry." This is a big one in weight loss programs. If you are, in fact, hungry, eat something on plan and nutritious.

Anger or agitation is a big one since you're probably a member of polite society. Being angry or just a little agitated isn't bad. What tends to lead to destructive behavior (like raging on your kids) is an inability to express this anger. If you are angry, yelling or inhaling all the chips and salsa in the world won't help you. This is a good time to take a walk, talk to someone and vent, or do anything else to get this angry energy out. You need an emotional and possibly even physical release for this anger. Use it to your advantage.

When you don't feel your best, physically or emotionally, the tendency for many is to hide away. **Loneliness** can sneak up on you. Even when surrounded by people all day, you can still feel lonely and like you're not making meaningful connections. Remember, being alone isn't the same as loneliness. Loneliness is an emptiness that you may try to fill with food, sleep, or even alcohol. If you are feeling lonely, try to reach out to family, a friend, or even someone on social media. Simple human contact can begin to fill the hole you feel inside.

As far as being **tired**, it is just a fact of life for many women. This is where you will need to listen to your body and use your good sense. Are you not working out because you're legitimately tired, or are you feeling a little lazy or just don't want to? Fatigue can be a big problem when you're trying to eat healthy food. I know that my biggest problem with avoiding comfort foods, delivery food, and other junk is being tired. You simultaneously want to have something easy and something comforting. You begin to crave high-fat, high-calorie foods because your body is seeking energy. Your best options are to have a snack with protein or just to take a nap or go to bed.

The goal of the HALT method and noting your associations between behaviors and emotions is to ensure that you're acting for healthy and effective reasons.

Cognitive Behavior Therapy (CBT)

As you embark on your plan toward a new healthy lifestyle, there may be a need to work on your attitudes and beliefs along with your actual behaviors and emotions. Cognitive Behavior Therapy (CBT) is a method where you're essentially your own therapist (cool, right?) and you take a solution-focused approach to solve problems and learn the skills you need to make adjusting to your new lifestyle easier. The goal of CBT is to help you change your thinking and behaviors and then to keep them that way. This method has been demonstrated to be wildly effective since Dr. Aaron T. Beck developed it back in the 1960s.

CBT is a practical, use-anywhere approach to problem solving. Its goal is to assist you in changing your patterns of thinking or behavior that are behind your challenges and difficulties by changing the way you feel and respond emotionally to situations (7). CBT focuses on the thoughts, images, attitudes, and beliefs that relate to the way you behave. For example, there is an underlying reason why you overreact when stressed or avoid your friends when you feel overwhelmed.

We all have a constant internal dialogue that affects how we act and react. Within this dialogue, we have what Beck referred to as automatic thoughts, which are emotion-filled and sometimes completely undetected by our conscious thinking.

Through CBT skills, you can learn to identify, become aware of, and alter these automatic thoughts into those that are more beneficial to reaching your goals and living a happy, healthy life.

When we don't identify and recognize these types of thoughts, we can get stuck in a pattern of unhelpful thinking, or worse, base our thinking on incorrect and irrational thoughts. For example, if one of your automatic thoughts is, "Everyone will stare at me at the gym. I'm not fit enough to go there yet," you will then operate based on the belief that you're either "not ready" to start a fitness plan or that you aren't someone who could fit in if you did. This error-based thinking leads to other misguided beliefs, like, "If I could just work out, I would lose weight. I can't work out because people will stare, so I'll never lose weight." Spiraling on and on and on, these thoughts can grow a life of their own and create your whole world around you. This leads to making the original thought an even bigger deal than it needs to be and leaving you stuck. Many of our stressful episodes come from this process of focusing on automatic thoughts that are destructive. We build and build based on a negative thought and make ourselves unhappy for no good reason.

There are three skill areas needed to put the brakes on your destructive automatic thoughts and to adjust your thought patterns:

- Awareness
- Questioning
- Challenging

When something happens or is going to happen—an event, a decision, something in your environment—you will have automatic thoughts contributing to your internal dialogue. When you have these thoughts, emotions are attached. When the emotions are negative, you are more likely to have a tendency to assume that the outcome of what is happening will be negative. Sometimes this is an accurate assessment. If you're about to drive into a tornado, you can assume the outcome will be bad. We are not looking to change your innate sense of self-preservation in terms of outcomes. The goal of being aware of your thoughts is simply knowing that they are there and identifying the emotions associated with them.

After becoming aware of the thoughts and evaluating the associated emotions, you need to question this emotional response. Is this an accurate assessment? Is this a rational thought? Can this thought be cast in a more positive light? Questioning allows you to take the time to evaluate your response and decide if it's appropriate for the situation.

If you find that your thoughts and emotions may not be the most appropriate for the situation at hand, you should challenge those thoughts and try to find a more effective way to respond to the situation. You can mentally weigh the possible outcomes, you can write a pros and cons list, you can even step through some thought experiments on how different responses would work out.

As you become more experienced with being aware of, questioning, and challenging your thoughts, you will become very adept at moving your thinking and reactions toward those that are more in line with your goals and how you want to interact with the world. You'll be able to put the brakes on destructive thoughts and the out-of-control spiraling that comes from them.

Here are some specific ways you can work through the CBT process to align your thought process with your goals and save yourself some grief:

Actively challenge your beliefs, attitudes, and thoughts by asking these questions:

- What would I tell my best friend if she were in this same situation?
- Am I overgeneralizing?
- Am I assuming the worst-case scenario will happen?
- What is the worst thing that could happen?
- What is a best-case scenario?
- Is this situation within my control?
- Is there any way to look at this in a positive light?
- Will this matter next week, next month, or next year?

You can also use the **ABCD process** if you're having an especially hard time. This thought identification exercise is a way for us to match thoughts, feelings, and events. We typically address problems first in our thinking, but this method actually has you approach the thought backwards by addressing the outcome first. Like the questions above, this process will slow you down so you can think and reason before you let your emotions carry you away.

The A stands for **Activating Event**. This is what is happening or what you anticipate happening. For example, "I am going out to eat at a restaurant I've never been to."

B stands for **Belief/Thought**. This includes your thoughts associated with the event. In this example, you may think, "I have no idea what I can eat that is on my plan! I'll be tempted by the bread basket and desserts. I'll be forced to eat something bad for me because everyone else will, or they'll think I'm weird if I'm eating healthy." You can begin to see that some of these thoughts are irrational and could be easily controlled or reframed as positive.

C stands for **Consequence**. What are the emotional or behavioral consequences of this event? For this example, they may be anxiety, stress, fear, or lack of self-control. By completing the ABC part of this process, you can identify what thoughts are "real" concerns, what thoughts can be reframed or avoided, and what may actually need your attention. When your thoughts don't exactly fit with the facts, you can spin yourself up into a frenzy worrying over something that is less significant than you thought before.

Finally, D—**Dispute**. This is where you question and challenge the thoughts you've become aware of in A, B, and C. You will add evidence and facts that dispute the thoughts you've encountered in the ABCD process, and you'll work to find a way around the problems and emotional fallout you've noticed in this process. It's critical to deliberately dispute each thought, and if it is irrational or unhelpful, to turn it around to one that will get you through the situation and toward your goals.

In your dispute, put yourself in the place of an objective advice giver. If your best friend came to you with the event and thoughts you listed above, how would you respond to her? For our example, I would say, "Going to a restaurant I've never been to is less of an issue these days now that most places post a menu online. If they don't happen to have one up, I'll brainstorm what foods most places have that I can make work for me. Most restaurants have salads and some grilled chicken or fish. I can ask them to prepare the meal either without a sauce or other element that makes it outside my plan. I could also eat a snack before going out so I'm not starving. If a bread basket comes, I'll plan that into my daily meal, or, I can ignore it and get a starter salad or a soup. I don't have to tell anyone I'm on a diet. Even if someone asks, is it a big deal? I can just say I'm trying to eat light tonight. Would I think my friends were weird if they were on diets or were eating light? No, so why would they feel that way? No one is in control of my dinner besides me. I won't be forced into eating anything I don't want to. This dinner is supposed to be fun."

See how challenging your thoughts can make you see things more rationally? In life, you'll find yourself hitting roadblocks and times of discomfort. Don't let yourself get stressed out! I challenge you to stop for a moment and be aware of what is going on. Address your thoughts and feelings and make them work for you.

Okay, so you've learned about being mindful. You've also learned to halt and assess your feelings and to stop the pattern of destructive automatic thoughts. All of this requires your attention. The unwritten step that we need to take before working on self-awareness is actually learning to pay more attention—to our thoughts, bodies, environments, relationships—to everything. As with your emotional intelligence, your attention skills can be improved with practice.

Begin by paying attention to what's happening around you right now. Notice how you feel emotionally. Take a deep breath and notice how your body feels. The more you can be attentive, self-aware, and mindful, the more control you have over your lifestyle. This puts you in the position to accomplish anything you want. With attention, you can cultivate the ability to focus and be as effective as possible. The bottom line is: If you don't have your full attention on a task or goal, you will not be as effective as you could be in reaching that goal. And you'll be totally stressed out.

Self-Care and Relaxation

One of the primary ways to combat daily stress is with regular self-care. We're going to start our self-care and relaxation in an unlikely place—your surroundings. When your surroundings are chaotic, it's easy to feel chaotic inside. The piles of things to get to and lists of things to do are fine . . . if you're doing them within a day or so. Otherwise, they become reminders of all that is on your plate and become a constant stressor. If you can't take care of those piles or items on your list right away, organize them the best you can and put them out of sight. The clearer, cleaner, and calmer your surroundings are, the less you are going to feel overwhelmed; the less overwhelmed we feel, the less likely we are to reach for an unhealthy snack or skip a workout.

When our environment is clear, we automatically feel relieved. That relief is necessary to truly relax because seeing that stack of things you need to handle keeps you in a stressed state. Relaxation is a process that decreases the effects of stress on your mind and body. By using relaxation techniques to calm yourself and refocus your attention, you can better deal with everyday stress as well as the stress related to making a big change like you are now. Even simple relaxation techniques can reduce physical and mental stress symptoms. Our lives are already full and hectic, so we need to be deliberate about our relaxation time. We have input from people, our environments, our phone, computers, tablets, and on and on. This keeps us in a constant state of alertness—so much that we begin to feel stressed and overworked, leading us to be tired, unhappy, impatient, and even depressed.

This constant state of alertness takes a toll on our overall health, and often the fallout is seen across our lives and in our bodies. Having a little time to yourself is critical for your health and well-being. You can take this time in a variety of ways, including (but not at all limited to) meditating, doing breathing exercises, journaling, doing an active meditation like progressive relaxation, knitting, practicing yoga, dancing, walking, or even just taking a few breaks over the course of the day to stop and be at peace. In this section, I'll tell you about some different ways you can carve out quiet time for yourself.

It may seem like your life is so full and cramped that there isn't time for meditation or even time for yourself. In fact, meditation actually makes you more efficient and gives you more time by calming and focusing your mind as well as helping you understand your own mind, body, and processes. Meditation is really just time for you to be still and content. Even the still part isn't necessary! Learning to relax will make you more efficient in your everyday life. Meditation will: increase your feeling of being calm, improve your interaction with others, teach you to slow down and not try to do multiple things at once, and focus your attention on what you are doing at any given time.

Meditation can be done in a variety of ways, and there is no wrong way to meditate. You can sit cross-legged and close your eyes, you can lie down, you can have your eyes open, you can even be doing something like knitting, coloring, or walking. Your goal with meditation is to let the outside world fall away and to journey inward. Your focus is on quieting your mind, so if sitting still isn't your thing, the repetitive motion of a stationary bike or beading a necklace can help you take your mind off of everything external.

Meditation will train your mind to become less responsive to stress and will result in physiological changes that counteract the harmful effects of stress throughout the day. One possible goal of meditation, no matter what technique you use, can be to find a way for you not to diffuse the thoughts you find disturbing. You can do this by focusing your attention on something that has no emotional value to you. Oftentimes, it's the disturbing thoughts that activate your stress.

To avoid stress, you will want to train your mind to briefly clear itself from disturbing thoughts. When you are trying to relax your mind and an intrusive thought enters, focusing your attention on a word, phrase, sound, or repetitive movement helps you to let go temporarily of the invading thought. To get the full benefits from meditation, you must practice and repeat the techniques. The more you practice relaxing your mind, the easier and more effective it will become.

I'll give you an example of one type of meditation technique. Sit in a comfortable position. Close your eyes and breathe deeply. Let your breathing be slow and relaxed. Focus all your attention on your breathing. Notice your chest and abdomen moving in and out. Block out all other thoughts, feelings, and sensations. If you feel your attention wandering, bring it back to your breathing. As you inhale, imagine the word "peace;" as you exhale, say the word "calm." Draw out the pronunciation of the word in your head so it lasts for the entire breath, like p-e-e-e-a-a-a-a-c-c-c-e-e-e and c-a-a-a-l-l-l-m-m-m. Repeat these words in your head as you breathe to help you concentrate. Continue the exercise until you feel very relaxed.

Another meditation technique is focusing, which can be done anywhere for any amount of time. To practice focusing, select a small personal object you like. Focus all your attention on this object as you inhale and exhale slowly and deeply for one to two minutes. While you are doing the exercise, try not to let any other thoughts or feelings enter your mind. If they do, just return your attention to the object. At the end of this exercise, you will probably feel more peaceful and calmer. Any tension or nervousness you were feeling upon starting the exercise should be diminished.

Guided imagery is used for relaxation and it helps to create a sense of peace. It involves creating mental pictures that calm you down and relax your mind. There are plenty of guided meditations on YouTube and other websites. These recordings will allow you to focus fully on listening and being still instead of trying to come up with what you should focus on by yourself. These guided meditations can be especially helpful on days when you are overwhelmed and need help quieting your mind.

If you don't have access to guided recordings where you are, you can do this on your own. Choose a setting that is calming to you, whether a tropical beach, a favorite childhood spot, or even sitting on your balcony. Close your eyes and let your worries drift away. Imagine your restful place. Picture it as vividly as you can—everything you can see, hear, smell, and feel. Guided imagery works best if you incorporate as many sensory details as possible.

Meditation can be used not only to increase your focus and calm your mind during the day, but it can be used to help you relax and prepare to sleep. Progressive muscle relaxation is a relaxation technique involving the systematic tensing and relaxing of muscle groups. To do it, lie down in a comfortable position. Allow your arms to rest at your sides. Inhale and exhale slowly and deeply. Clench your hands into fists and hold them tightly for 15 seconds. As you do this, relax the rest of your body. Visualize your fists contracting, becoming tighter and tighter. Then let your hands relax. On relaxing, see a golden light flowing into the entire body, making all your muscles soft and pliable.

Now, tense and relax the following parts of your body in this order: face, shoulders, back, stomach, pelvis, legs, feet, and toes. Hold each part tensed for 15 seconds and then relax your body for 30 seconds before going on to the next part. Finish the exercise by shaking your hands and imagining the remaining tension flowing out of your fingertips. If you like, you can also do this at your desk, on the subway, in the car—anywhere. Just change "lie down" to "sit" and you're ready to relax.

Breathing exercises are an especially helpful tool you can use anywhere to relax in a flash. Deep breathing is such a simple, yet powerful, relaxation technique. It's easy to learn, can be practiced almost anywhere, and provides a quick way to get your stress levels in check. Deep breathing is the cornerstone of many other relaxation practices, too, and can be combined with other relaxing elements such as music. Here's how to practice deep breathing:

- Sit comfortably with your back straight.
- Put one hand on your chest and the other on your stomach.

- Breathe in through your nose.
- The hand on your stomach should rise.
- The hand on your chest should move very little.
- Exhale through your mouth, pushing out as much air as you can while contracting your abdominal muscles.
- The hand on your stomach should move in as you exhale, but your other hand should move very little.
- Continue to breathe in through your nose and out through your mouth.
- Try to inhale enough so that your lower abdomen rises and falls.
- Count slowly as you exhale.

Once you've done this enough to know what it feels like for you to take deep breaths, you won't need to use your hands on your chest and stomach, so you can practice anywhere, anytime.

Another option for relaxation is writing. Writing your thoughts about things that are troubling you can help with not only reducing the stress you're feeling, but also for preventing future stress from building up. Try writing continuously for a few minutes and work up to longer periods. You can pretend you are writing to a friend, or family member, or even to the person who is stressing you out. Write what you feel. If you run out of things to say, just repeat what you have already written. I want you to let go of detail to grammar, spelling, or sentence structure and avoid censoring or editing your words. Just write the thoughts that appear in your mind. Don't read anything that you have written while you're still writing. Throw away your writing when you are finished, or keep it in your journal. Whatever feels best.

Humor is also a wonderful stress reducer. It is clinically proven to be effective in combating stress, although the exact mechanism is not known. Experts say a good laugh relaxes tense muscles, speeds more oxygen into your system, and lowers your blood pressure. One way to do this is to watch a funny movie or TV show. You can also watch videos on YouTube, listen to a funny podcast, watch stand-up comedy, or look at a humorous website.

Finally, if you're feeling antsy from your stress or you're just not one for sitting still, you can try meditative movement. It can be slow movement like tai chi or yoga, or more active like dance or weight lifting. I enjoy walking, and it seems to cure everything for me. It also boosts creativity and helps you figure out problems.

What's important here isn't how you relax and care for yourself, it's just that you do it. Experiment with some of these ideas for relaxation and make caring for yourself a priority to keep stress from ruining your life.

Support System

A support system is important for stress relief because it provides you with people to talk to and an outlet for blowing off steam. Just about everything is easier when you have support. Let's take a few minutes to think about the kinds of support you need to be as successful as possible, and then consider who might be able to give it to you.

List as many people or sources as you can think of. These may be unconventional forms of support, too, like your new puppy who loves walks or an online group of people from all over the world.

The three major areas you'll need support in are emotional support, practical support, and information support. Emotional support involves having people who can listen when you need someone to talk to. These people are also important as you make changes in this program. They can encourage you to keep going when you're feeling frustrated and celebrate your successes. They don't have to be trying to achieve goals alongside you, but that type of person may also be of great support. Be open to who can support you in tough times and to who can help make reaching your goals a little more pleasant along the way.

Some possible sources of emotional support are your partner, relatives, friends, coworkers, and online buddies you meet through social media. Maybe there's a local meetup for runners or hikers or aspiring cooks, or others you can connect with.

Practical support comes from people or other sources that can help you with tips, logistics, and other needs that directly relate to making life easier for meeting your goals. These are people to exercise or shop for healthy foods with, swap cooking ideas and recipes with, or even help with occasional child care or home chores on extra-busy days. This kind of support can also come from outsourcing and automating parts of your life to save yourself time, like hiring a maid, getting a Roomba, having groceries delivered, and other conveniences.

Some possible sources are your partner, relatives, friends, coworkers, others with similar goals, service companies, apps, and products that make what you do simpler. I want to stress that getting help is not a sign of failure. Doing it all for no reason isn't a good look.

Finally, you will need support in the form of information to help you make decisions, eliminate uncertainty, stay emotionally healthy, and for general problem-solving. Friends who have dealt with similar situations, books, online groups—all are good options. For support with living a healthy lifestyle, information can come from doctors and health professionals (including registered dietitians, personal trainers, physical therapists, counselors, and health coaches), health organization websites, organized groups, and reputable books and magazines.

When it comes to finding health information, though, be very careful to vet your sources. I can't let you go without a little lecture on smart information sourcing. Make sure you are finding your information from certified and credible professionals and websites that are affiliated with respected medical organizations. For example, the Mayo Clinic's advice will be far more trustworthy than something you found on Pinterest or a mommy message board.

Once you've realized what you need and who can help you, start connecting the dots. Ask your designated supporters if they're willing to help—and if so, talk about how they can support you. If you don't have a support team, create one. We all want to feel supported, right? Don't be afraid to invite them along for a walk, dance class, or trip to a healthy restaurant you want to check out.

Recognize the importance of give-and-take, and don't forget the many other parts of your life that aren't stressful. No one, and I mean no one, wants to sit around and hear all about your troubles without some reciprocity and a break from complaints. Express your appreciation for their support, and be ready to return the favor and help others.

PILLAR SEVEN: ENERGY MANAGEMENT

"I Just Can't"

I interviewed women while doing research for this book, and I was overwhelmed by how many of them said that their biggest health concern was not having energy. Some of them put it in more colorful terms, like "my body is shutting down from stress," "I feel worse than when I was up all night with a newborn," "I've actually face-planted on my keyboard from tiredness," and "I try to do things after work, but I just can't. I've lost the will to be social." I hadn't expected this to be the most talked-about health issue, but I should have. I feel it too. I think my best friends are those who don't make me leave my house or put on pants to hang out.

There has been an explosion of think pieces lately on why women are so burned out. This burnout has become normal, but in this case, normal doesn't mean right. We take on work, home, and social lives. We're constantly connected to others on our phones, tablets, and computers, and it's the growing expectation that we remain so available. Women often come home from work to do what is referred to as the "second shift," where they handle household chores and childcare after a full day.

As we've optimized our lives with smart homes, electronic personal assistants, quick shipping, and productivity apps out the wazoo, we haven't used that saved time and effort to relax and recharge. We see it as an opportunity to do and add more.

All About Energy

If only there were more hours in the day, we would be happier, healthier, and more content.

Time is the problem. Or is it? When you stop and really think about it, you'll probably find that you do have the time. If you don't have any time, how is it that you managed to watch an entire series on Netflix recently? That is literally an entire day you managed to squeeze in. Okay, so maybe you actually do have time.

If you're like most women, the problem is energy. The reason you crash out in the evenings is because you have no energy after a tough day at work. Weekends are a bust because you can't bring yourself to tackle your growing to-do list. Many of us have chronically low energy. We're so focused on achieving and getting things done that we never stop to consider that our energy levels perhaps aren't what they should be, or that we could do a lot to feel better.

The first thing you need to understand about managing your energy levels is that energy begets energy. On the other hand, if you go about energy management in the wrong way or you don't think about it properly, your low energy will only get worse. Let's say you wake up in the morning with zero energy. So, you hit snooze too many times, rush out the door stressed, get to work, work slowly and accomplish little to nothing, come home late and stressed, get dinner delivery, and then go to bed late. After that awful day, you're actually going to have even less energy tomorrow, and the cycle repeats.

Even on your best days, you won't have a steady state of high energy. When managing your energy, consider that you will always have natural ebbs and flows because of your body's rhythms. We're all different, so pay attention to the changes in your energy levels. Note your energy level every couple of hours throughout the day. The trick is to learn your own ebbs and flows and then, rather than fight them, to embrace them and use them to your advantage.

Your energy isn't infinite, so your daily priorities should be based on what you have the energy for rather than what fits into your schedule. Sometimes you'll have to say no to certain things, and it'll be hard. You'll probably have trouble rationalizing this change at first since you're used to basing your day on time rather than energy. But, as you start to feel better and use your energy more wisely, you'll be able to say yes to more of what you want to.

Because your energy is finite, it is also smart to make sure that you aren't wasting energy in your routine by doing things that aren't necessary or that could be made easier. This will not only increase your energy, but it will reduce your stress.

The Myth of Doing it All

The modern woman wears busyness as a badge of honor. There was even a book and then a movie with Sarah Jessica Parker called *I Don't Know How She Does It*. That archetype of the superwoman who juggles work, family, social life, and community with grace and skill is an impossible standard. Gee, I wonder why you feel so tired all the time?

I challenge you to break free from the myth of doing it all and start seeing ease, flow, and calm as the ideal. If you could let go of what everyone else thinks of you and what you *should* be doing, you'll likely find that your energy doesn't deplete so easily. This goes for everyone—the stay at home moms, single gals, working women, and ladies of all ages.

What weighs you down differs by your situation, but it isn't always the big things. Sometimes it's "death by a thousand cuts," where it's the overload of trivial tasks that eventually becomes too much. Adding just one more little thing and packing your schedule to the brim leads to stress and overwhelm. It's also a big reason why you might have low energy and don't know why. It's "just" laundry. It's "just" an extra hour at work. It's "just" one favor you have to drive across town to do. Individually, is each thing difficult? Nope. That's where many of us get into trouble. We feel guilty for feeling tired and run down since when we start listing what we have to do, no one task or obligation is a big deal. The big deal is the accumulation of these things. And, yes, your feelings about overwhelm, fatigue, and low energy are very real and very valid.

I'm going to say that again, your tiredness is real and valid. Brushing it aside and thinking you're being weak or dramatic doesn't help anything. You are not built to do it all. Though you're awesome, you're still human and don't need to take on the world.

This section is a little bit of tough love, but someone needs to stop you from slowly killing yourself in the name of doing just one more little thing. Not only is doing it all a myth, so is the sister of it, the myth that women can have it all. There will always be sacrifices with our time and needs, but we absolutely cannot continue to achieve and grow and be who we want to be if we sacrifice health. That lack of energy is a sign of your health sacrifices.

Busyness has become the new normal for most of us. There is personal satisfaction, but there's also social pressure to do and have it all. You have to protect your health and set limits in your life and stick to them. Sheryl Sandberg, author of *Lean In*, addresses the myth of doing it all and the guilt many women feel when they sacrifice family for their careers. But, this advice applies to all of you. Sandberg says that "guilt management is as important as time management." Your guilt and constant need to take on everything is moderately helping others and majorly hurting you. This isn't to say that you should be selfish and not do favors—of course you should! What I'm saying is that the guilt that forces you to do everything and take on even more is a problem.

Setting aside any guilt you may feel, I'd like you to focus instead on defining what success means for your and your life. In other words, if you were on your deathbed, what would you like to have done with your life? Be specific about the indicators of success. What are some of the big milestones you want to hit for success, like a graduate degree, owning a home, having kids, and donating a significant amount of time or money to your favorite charity. Those are just some ideas, and yours will probably be different.

Your definition is not at all about what success means to others close to you or in society. It's what is important to you in the big picture. Once you do this, I'll bet you won't have written down never taking your full vacation time at work, being the best 3rd grade room mother in history, or even having the world's cleanest house. This definition and your milestones will be deeply personal and unique to you. This should be your personal vision statement for life. If your daily activities don't lead you toward that vision, consider if you need them at all. We can't live in a bubble, so you can't jettison all responsibilities, but you can prioritize and use your energy in a smart way.

To go back to Sheryl Sandberg for a moment, she also gave this piece of advice, "Success is making the best choices we can ... and accepting them." Your energy is limited, so don't spend it on guilt or worry about your choices. Here are some other things I'd like you to consider doing.

Decide what really matters in life. This will likely be what aligns with your definition of success or what creates the most good in your life or someone else's. Be energy-efficient and focus on the big stuff.

Along with doing what matters most, I'd like you to also make peace with occasionally dropping the ball. If you want to preserve your energy, you can't do everything. When you get what matters done, what's left is less important. It's okay to take those things off your list or move them to another day when you're refreshed.

I know you're probably the go-to gal, but be willing to ask people for help. This help can be from family members, friends, or anyone else who would feel perfectly comfortable asking for help from you. You're not an endless fount of energy, so let others take some of the burden.

Finally, a big goal should be learning how to be comfortable with saying no to the things you don't need to or want to do. You can still be a generous, caring, in-charge person and say no sometimes. We all have limits. Knowing yours and sticking to them is a big step in finding a healthy lifestyle filled with both energy and meaning.

Sleep

While you may be tempted to go, go, go during this program, like you're probably doing in the rest of your life, you must remember that your body needs rest to recover from not only your exercise routine, but also your daily routine and stressors. Sleep is when your body restores and repairs itself. Not allowing for this recovery time can lead to multiple health issues, including susceptibility to added stress and possibly weight gain. This weight gain doesn't all come from evil unseen forces that come along when you don't sleep. Some of it comes from consuming extra calories because you are awake. Even more, people who stay up late tend to consume a higher number of calories from fat than they would otherwise during daytime hours.

Researchers have found that the subjects who spent only four hours in bed from 4 a.m. to 8 a.m. for five consecutive nights gained more weight than those who were in bed for 10 hours each night from 10 p.m. to 8 a.m. Does this mean you're doomed to gain weight if you're a night owl or don't sleep much? No, of course not. This is simply a factor to consider as you are on this mission to create optimal health and make your body more efficient.

Good health is complicated and depends on multiple factors—diet, daily activity, stress, social support from friends and family, attitudes, beliefs, access to healthy food, socioeconomic status, and on and on. The purpose of this program is to help you live your best and healthiest life. This best life includes adequate rest and sleep.

Unless you are very disciplined or are unlike the majority of people, you likely do not get enough sleep. Here are some reasons why you may be short on quality sleep.

First, your bedroom probably isn't optimal for sleeping. Making your bedroom a sweet-dreams zone is the first step in ensuring that you are getting quality sleep. Your room should be dark, cool, and quiet. You should also be aware of your comfort and set yourself up for success by having a comfortable mattress and bed linens.

Next, you might be overstimulated. Does your mind race up to and past bedtime? It's hard for most of us to silence our brains and get into a restful state of mind. Reduce the biological reasons for restless sleep by cutting yourself off from caffeine after lunchtime. You may also be pumping your brain with energizing endorphins if you work out in the evening. Begin to think about the effects of your habits on bedtime by midday. Experiment a little with your caffeine intake and timing of exercise.

Third, you may snore or have sleep apnea. People with a history of snoring or waking up feeling tired and generally unrested may be candidates for a sleep study to diagnose a possible sleep disorder, such as sleep apnea—pauses in your breathing while you sleep. If you've had a history of non-restful sleep or if you have a history of snoring, talk to your doctor. Sleep apnea is easily treatable, but when left untreated has been linked to several health conditions, including high blood pressure, heart disease, and type-2 diabetes.

Finally, chronic stress might have made you deficient in melatonin. Melatonin is the most important hormone when it comes to helping you fall asleep and stay asleep. Chronic stress can deplete your melatonin (among other horrors). Luckily, melatonin supplements are readily available and simple to try. If you are interested in supplements, start with 1-3 milligrams and increase the dosage as needed.

I'm going to bet that you want to know how to get more sleep and make it more worthwhile. This list is simple, but it may take some time to change your habits and have your body cooperate, so be patient with yourself. Some tips that most researchers agree on are:

- Using your bed for only sleep and sex
- Limiting naps and using them wisely when you do take them (more on that coming up)
- Avoiding caffeine after noon
- Avoiding liquids close to bedtime
- Turning off electronics at least 30 minutes before bed
- Keeping the same bedtime and wake time.
- Getting regular exercise—but not late in the evening

Most importantly, if you have a sleepless night, don't panic or perseverate over it. Doing so will increase your anxiety and make it even harder to fall asleep. If you are unable to sleep after 15 minutes of lights-out time, get up and do something else until you're tired. Reading or watching TV in another room, working on a craft project, or anything else that lets you relax is perfect. Try again once you feel tired.

We're going to end our discussion on sleep with a run-through of tips that go beyond your nightly rest.

Your day starts best when you have a good morning. Part of that is getting out of bed and getting the day started. I know it can be hard to wake up, and you may need extreme alarm noises to make it happen, but try to wake up as gently as you can. Waking up startled gets you into a panicked state right away. That panic uses energy, which means you have less for the rest of the day. Find an alarm setting on your phone or an alarm clock that will ease you into the day.

I'd like you to also resist hitting snooze. Doing so doesn't really help you anyway, since you're getting poor sleep at best in those 9 minutes of snooze. If you have to, position your alarm so you actually have to get out of bed to turn it off—and then don't crawl back in bed! Use the time you would have snoozed to wake yourself up with a few stretches or thinking through your day.

During the day, you may feel a little sleepy. I have two thoughts on naps. First, if you are having trouble sleeping at night or didn't get enough sleep, don't nap. Go to bed earlier and make up your sleep then. If you slept fine and you're just feeling like a nap would be nice, use power naps. These work especially well when your brain is on overload from working, studying, or emotions.

I promised I'd get back to how to use naps effectively! Well, studies by the National Institute of Mental Health found that a 60-minute power nap can not only reverse the effects of information overload, it may also help us better retain what we have learned. And that's on top of the rest you get.

Now we've reached the end of the day, and it's time to set yourself up for a good night. If you have trouble getting to bed on time, set a sleep-time alarm. I told you that it's important to stick to a sleep schedule, and this is a good way to make sure it happens. Set your alarm such that you have time to wind down before bedtime. About 30 minutes to an hour before lights out works. During that time, do some deep breathing in bed or meditate for five to 10 minutes to clear your mind and help you get to a restful place. Another tip is to set the thermostat to a cooler temperature when the alarm goes off. Sleeping in cooler temperatures leads to better sleep. If you can stand it, try 65 degrees.

Why are You So Tired?

Let's take a look at why you feel tired, even if you are getting adequate rest and are otherwise healthy. I would like you to figure out why you are tired. Choose a few representative days and write down all that you do, big and small. Consider what took the most energy to do. Include how you felt at the end of each day. This worksheet is also in the free program workbook on my website at www.tsirona.com/ybbbook (see the QR code in the Introduction).

We're going to get some more information on why you may be tired. For 1-2 weeks, track how long you sleep at night. You can also track your naps if you like. Make some notes on how you feel when you wake up. Are you rested? Will you positively die if you don't hit snooze? This worksheet is also in the free program workbook on my website at www.tsirona.com/ybb-book (see the QR code in the Introduction).

Staying Energized During the Day

The biggest health complaint I hear from my clients is that they're lacking energy. They talk about dropping into bed at night, absolutely exhausted from the day. Many have even given up hobbies and things they used to find fun, like reading or watching TV after work, because of being so tired. This is a factor you can handle—I promise.

Though it's my clients' most-discussed problem, I don't address it first in this book. It's in one of the last sections because your energy is a result of your lifestyle—most importantly your nutrition, activity, and stress management. And this will likely be a stubborn issue, because you'll need to have gotten your healthy lifestyle going for a little while to see long-term changes in your energy. Be patient. It's coming.

There are some things you can do to help your energy along while your healthy habits are taking hold. First, it's important to know there are three types of energy that you are using each day: mental, emotional, and physical. Mental energy is used for ideas and thinking—it's what you've used up when you're exhausted from a long day of sitting at your desk working. Emotional energy is used for your feelings, and it can get drained when you are dealing long-term with powerful emotions like sadness, fear, and excitement. Emotional energy can get depleted after having lunch with a friend who is leaning on you for support. Physical energy is what we think of most when talking about energy levels. It's what we use for body movement, like exercise and activity. All three types of energy are important to look after, and a depletion of any one of these can lead to fatigue. The tips I'm giving you in this chapter will address all three types of energy, since you want to feel like all three tanks are full enough to be healthy.

Our first stop in an energy discussion is caffeine, since it's probably your secret for morning pep or solution for an afternoon slump. If you are not sensitive to caffeine, it is perfectly fine for you to consume it. In fact, it even has benefits. Studies have found that caffeine helps boost memory and reduces the risk of Parkinson's. Even more interesting, studies have found that frequent low doses of caffeine, about a quarter cup of coffee, were more effective than a few larger doses of caffeine in keeping people alert. You can reap those benefits by nursing your coffee through to lunchtime instead of guzzling.

But the most appropriate response to feeling fatigued is to drink water. When you are low on fluids, your body's first signal is fatigue. On the topic of getting enough fluids, you can also try herbal teas in hot or iced forms. Though I doubt you're taking liquid lunches very often, remember that lunchtime alcohol has a sedative effect and will make you tired mid-afternoon. Same goes for happy hour. Be careful with alcohol if you want to have energy afterward.

You will also want to use food strategically to keep your energy at optimal levels all day. For energy management, it's better to eat small meals and snacks every few hours than three large meals a day to give your brain a steady supply of nutrients. If you can't swing that with your schedule, it's not a deal-breaker, so don't stress. You can get most of the benefit by making sure you don't skip meals and by having a snack that combines protein, a little fat and some fiber, like peanut butter on a whole-wheat cracker or some cheese with an ounce of nuts.

Speaking of what to eat, you'll want to opt for high-energy food, like fruits, vegetables, nuts and seeds, quality cuts of meat, dairy, and whole grains. Food with a low glycemic index —those whose sugars are absorbed slowly—may help you avoid the sugar crash after eating quickly absorbed sugars or refined starches. Foods with a low glycemic index include whole grains, high-fiber vegetables, nuts, and healthy oils— essentially, whole foods.

In general, high-carbohydrate foods have the highest glycemic indexes. Proteins and fats have glycemic indices that are close to zero. Eating a balanced diet can help ensure your vitamin, mineral, and nutrient needs are met and that, in turn, keeps you feeling energetic.

I want you to pay special attention to a few things, though. First, your magnesium. This mineral is used in over 300 biochemical reactions in your body, and when levels are even a little low, your energy can drop. To make sure you're getting enough, eat plenty of almonds, hazelnuts, Brazil nuts, cashews, walnuts, bran, dark leafy greens, and halibut.

Next, you need to get enough iron. An iron deficiency, called anemia, is a common cause of fatigue. Iron is essential for producing hemoglobin, which carries oxygen to your body's cells, where it is used to produce energy. Be sure to eat food with good sources of iron like red meat, green leafy vegetables, and dried beans.

Then there's B12. This vitamin helps make your DNA and your red blood cells, and it plays an important function in your nervous system. Since your body doesn't make vitamin B12, you have to get it from food or supplements—and frequently, since your body doesn't hold on to it for long. You can get your B12 from animal products like meat, fish, eggs, and milk, and from dried and fermented plant foods, such as tempeh.

Finally, you've likely heard you need Omega-3 fatty acids for preventing heart disease and lowering blood pressure, but they can also fight some of the symptoms of fatigue and low energy, like depression, bad mood, and poor memory. Excellent sources of Omega-3s are salmon, tuna, walnuts, flax seeds, leafy greens, and hemp seeds. You can also see about taking a supplement for your magnesium, iron, B12, and Omega-3s, but be sure to talk to your doctor first if you are on any medications.

I know the last thing you want to do when you're feeling low-energy is to exercise, but it could really help. Just 10 minutes of exercise is enough to get your blood pumping and increase oxygen flow to your brain and muscles. There's science behind this counterintuitive advice. Exercise gives your cells more energy to burn, circulates oxygen, and causes your body to release epinephrine and norepinephrine, stress hormones that in modest amounts can make you feel energized. It doesn't even have to be anything hard or sweaty. A walk around the block is a good start. When you get moving, the boost in energy is usually immediate and lasts at least an hour. But, keep it short and simple when you're doing this just to re-energize. Longer, more intense workouts will counteract this effect.

I've mentioned that stress is one of the biggest factors in draining our energy. I won't belabor this point, but I want to mention that stress-induced emotions consume huge amounts of your energy. Taking on just one more thing or saying yes to everyone steals your energy. One of the main reasons for fatigue is overwork, including professional, family, and social obligations. Lighten your load, and allow yourself some breathing room. You only get so much energy each day.

There are some simple lifestyle things you can do for a pick-me-up. Music has been proven to change your energy and uplift you. Listen to something with an upbeat tempo or that takes you back to good times. You can also practice gratitude to reinvigorate yourself. Even better, combine these practices with exercise, like a walk. This will flood your brain with happy neurotransmitters and endorphins. Magic!

Another way to get more focused on the positive and what matters is to do a digital detox. It's the only kind of detox I approve of. This could be for a day or, ideally, 30 days for anything besides the absolutely necessary, like work and your friends calling. Keep your device hidden. Read a book on the subway home. Take a look out the window. People watch while waiting for friends to arrive at dinner. Watch TV and only watch TV—no scrolling mindlessly while you do it. You'll find that you're more present and focused. That saves your energy for what matters.

Finally, make sure you get outside and get some sun and fresh air regularly. This is especially important in the winter. The natural light can improve your energy levels and help fight seasonal affective disorder—also known as the winter blahs. Try for 30 minutes to an hour outside.

Sometimes your lack of energy can have medical solutions. If you're constantly low on energy, ask your doctor about a blood test for thyroid dysfunction as well as anemia. Low thyroid function may be the cause of your fatigue, and it can be fixed easily with medication. Your thyroid functionality can become a problem for women after childbirth and often during perimenopause. Anemia, a reduction in red blood cells, leads to reduced oxygen flow to your organs. This reduction in red blood cells can mean your body isn't getting the level of oxygen necessary to sustain energy. There are many types of anemia, but the most common type is iron deficiency anemia, which is caused by a shortage of iron in your body. This type of anemia occurs in many pregnant women, but it can also be caused by heavy menstrual bleeding, an ulcer, and regular use of some over-the-counter pain relievers, especially aspirin. Iron deficiency anemia is also treated easily, this time through an iron supplement.

While many of you experience normal, expected fatigue from pushing too hard and doing too much, is it possible that you are experiencing chronic fatigue? Are you struggling to get through most days because you're exhausted? Are you tired before you've even done anything? The CDC says that between 1 and 4 million Americans have chronic fatigue syndrome, and that it's four times more common in women.

Chronic fatigue is extreme tiredness that doesn't improve with rest, and it often gets worse with physical or mental activity. It's severe, persistent fatigue, lasting six months or more and usually can't be explained by any underlying medical condition. You may have chronic fatigue if you experience four or more of these symptoms: memory or concentration issues, headaches, a sore throat, enlarged lymph nodes in your neck or armpits, unexplained muscle or joint pain, regularly unrefreshing sleep, or extreme exhaustion lasting more than 24 hours after physical or mental exercise.

If you're feeling tired all of the time and can't seem to shake it, you'll want to talk to your doctor. Don't panic, though. About 40 percent of people with symptoms I mentioned end up having a treatable condition like anemia, depression, stress, or thyroid issues.

Let's see what's going on throughout the day with your energy cycle. For 2-3 days, track your energy levels at these different times on a scale of one to five, with one being exhausted and five being fully energized:

- Waking up
- Mid-morning
- Lunchtime
- Mid-afternoon
- Dinnertime
- Bedtime

Where do you see dips? Peaks? Trends? This worksheet is also in the free program workbook on my website at www.t-sirona.com/ybbbook (see the QR code in the Introduction).

NOW WHAT?

Continued Motivation

Motivation is the biggest barrier between you and your goals, mostly because we expect motivation to do more than it can for us. No matter how motivated you are in the beginning, there will be times where you feel as if your motivation has ghosted you. We all get tired and bored or feel tempted to cheat on our goals. It might feel as though giving up on your goals and watching another season of a show is easier than making things happen now, but you'll regret giving up in the future.

Tracking is a proven way to stay motivated, but it's probably the first thing you'll be tempted to quit. Avoid that temptation. It's part of our nature to want to see results, and tracking will show you that you are making progress, however small. Because changes can be very subtle, or may not even show up in the mirror at first, it can be easy to get disheartened and think you're putting in all this work for nothing. When you keep track of everything, you have solid numbers to show that it's worth all the hard work you're putting in. Little successes add up to big changes, like a snowball rolling down a hill. You'll get a burst of excitement and motivation when you see results. But whatever you do, don't give up tracking, even if you're writing down every bit of that 3,000 calorie buffet you ate. Mistakes happen. Maybe it wasn't a mistake at all, and you just wanted to go nuts on a buffet once. It's cool. Write it down and move on, but avoid a chain reaction where you think, "Well, I ate an entire pizza, so what's the real harm in eating a sleeve of Thin Mints?"

Also be aware of social or environmental cues that seem to encourage undesired habits, and then manage those cues. For example, you may learn from tracking that you're more likely to overeat while watching TV, or whenever treats are out in the office, or when you're around a certain friend. Giving in to these cues can derail you quickly, since you're training yourself to react to those stimuli. We're not too far off from Pavlov's dog here.

You might then try changing the situation by separating the association of eating from the cue (don't eat while watching TV), avoiding or eliminating the cue (leave the office kitchen immediately after pouring coffee), or changing the circumstances surrounding the cue (plan to meet your friend in a non-food setting). In general, visible and reachable food items are often cues for unplanned eating. If it's hard to resist and it doesn't help you toward your goals, don't set yourself up for failure. Having these regular cues can kill your motivation.

Your goals are important to you, but it's easy to forget them or push them aside. Try writing your goals on post-it notes and putting them somewhere you can see them. This could be your refrigerator, your desk, your bathroom mirror or even as the background on your computer or phone. Seeing those goals every day will remind you why you're doing this in the first place. It could make you think twice when you're considering skipping your workout.

Although there is technically no best time to work out for health benefits, studies have shown that working out in the morning is better for your motivation. If you can get up and get your workout done right away, you'll feel like you've achieved something, and you'll give your motivation a boost for the rest of the day. It also gets things over with before you've even thought too much about it. The longer you leave it to fit in your workout, the better the chance some excuse will crop up to stop you from doing it. It's not like your day is suddenly going to free up later in most cases.

Use the support network you identified in the last section. Who or what can get you reset and back on track? Use these resources at the first sign of dying motivation. Having support and a little accountability will fix things right up.

Finally, make sure that your goals have doable tactics and that you have milestones and mini goals built into your plan. You may need to go back to the plan you wrote and break things down further. What's more motivational, a goal you'll reach in six months or multiple mini goals you can achieve in a week or two that all add up to the bigger goal? It's the mini goals. Success breeds success.

After Achieving a Goal

After achieving a big goal—or even multiple goals—it's time for a celebration . . . mostly. This point is also time for goal reassessment, possibly more education, new goals, and a slight tweak in your mindset. Something critically important for you to consider is how to set new goals and keep the momentum going.

You'll likely feel better physically, but you will see the biggest changes in your outlook and understanding of what it takes to set and achieve goals. If you have hit your short-term goals, you're probably ready to continue on, full steam ahead. If you have achieved your short- and long-term goals, it's time to focus on the long-term changes that will presumably last for the rest of your long, healthy life. This maintenance period is where things can get squirrely.

Resetting Goals

When you attain a goal, it's the perfect time for both reflection and a big appreciation of the lifestyle changes you made into habits to reach this point. You will now need to devise a plan to hang onto the habits that led to your success. You have reached a significant point on your path to wellness and in your healthy life. The problem is that attaining goals without knowing what you're aiming for next can be a major catalyst for demotivation. It's that "Now what?" feeling you get after accomplishing something significant and then feeling a hole left in your time, effort, and focus. It's like finishing a great TV or book series and feeling a little sad.

But, unlike a TV or book series, there is something next for you. There's always something else to aim for. Let's say you got the energy you hoped for, you're eating well, and you're being active on a daily basis. Maybe your next goal is to try a new type of exercise format or hike a certain trail. You could also make your next goal to recruit a friend to join you in your healthy lifestyle and help her make some changes. Your follow-on goals can be anything that builds on your successes.

To reset your goals, you can adjust current ones to be even more advanced or you can repeat the process in the Goal Setting pillar to set all new goals. To adjust a current goal to be more advanced, you could take the goal, "I will walk 10,000 steps per day every day until May 31st" and change it to, "I will walk 12,000 steps per day every day until December 31st." It can be that simple. Consider the exercise progressions discussed in the Movement pillar.

Perhaps this is the point where you're ready to commit to more meditation or quiet time or you would like to look into improving your sleep or even going on a yoga retreat. As in the beginning of this process, the sky's the limit for your goals!

If you want to repeat the process in this book, now is the time to get your SMART Goals Planner and Goals and Tactics Worksheet out to review your goals and plan. Read through them carefully and make any notes. As you are making notes and thinking about what your next goals will be, focus on your progress instead of focusing on what didn't work or what wasn't a good plan. Any small step forward counts. Maybe your progress was emotional or was an uptick in your confidence level. Maybe you're proud of trying something new or just getting through the goal-setting process. Make your new goals, tactics, and plans reflect what has worked for you and what you do well. Try to reduce the parts of your plan that didn't go as well as you thought or that you found clunky or unhelpful.

After writing down your thoughts on your last goals and plan, evaluate the following things about your plan:

- When you were focusing on these goals, where did your energy go? Did you spin your wheels?
- Did you feel like you were making progress that was worth the amount of work you put into it?
- What were your successes and proudest moments?
- What were your failures? Why did they happen?
- What do you wish you had done but didn't?
- What have you learned about yourself?
- What do you think you could improve?

Be completely honest with yourself. The more objectively you can evaluate your plan, the better you can do with setting your next group of goals and concocting those plans. Go through your SMART Goals Planner and Goals and Tactics

Worksheet and your notes one last time and use what you've learned to inform your next goals and plans. Be sure to take some time with the Resetting Goals and Making Workouts Harder worksheets when reevaluating goals. These will give you an idea of what will come next after you've completed your current goals.

FINAL THOUGHTS
CONCLUSION

You've come to the end of the book, but certainly not to the end of your journey. Health and wellness are determined by your daily actions, and what we've done here is align your healthy behaviors with your lifestyle and who you are so that it all flows together.

Creating a healthy lifestyle this way lets you put your health on autopilot. This leads to a feeling of ease and flow. If you don't feel it yet, you will soon. There is no right or wrong amount of time to have everything kick in, but I promise it will.

What you can look forward to with this naturally, easily healthy lifestyle is what psychologists call a flow state. This is when you're in the zone, everything comes together, and you feel blissfully in control. Nakamura and Csíkszentmihályi (8) found that these six things happen when you experience flow:

1. You have a focused concentration on the present moment. This might mean that you are mindful and tuned in to what is happening in the here and now rather than worrying about the past or future.

2. Your awareness and actions feel like they have merged so that you feel like you're moving and doing without needing to think. It's all natural and automatic.
3. You are not self-conscious, and you can put aside negative self-talk and worries.
4. You have a sense of personal control over your situation and what you are doing.
5. You are in such control and a state of ease that it's almost like time has slowed down and you can see and handle everything, like Neo in *The Matrix*.
6. You find that your healthy lifestyle isn't hard work that you hate to do. In fact, it's rewarding and something you end up liking!

This flow is your gift to yourself from the hard work you've done through this program. It's the reward you deserve! In this book, you've covered all of your bases and now you just need to keep following your plan until it's second nature. Then, you can set new goals if you want a challenge. Or not—it's up to you.

You have the power, the choice, and the ability to make your life any way you want it. Remember, you don't need to change everything to feel the impact on your health and happiness. Methodical, informed goal-setting, getting your mindset right, and getting out of your own way will lead to the healthy lifestyle you want, but you won't have to struggle with it constantly.

You are exactly where you are meant to be. You have the knowledge and the motivation. You have the brain power and the track record of success in the rest of your life. Just use it. I have a lot of faith in you.

TOOLS FROM KELLY

I want you to be healthy, happy, and crazy successful in your life, so I have multiple free resources for you:

- My blog with hundreds of posts on the pillars of a healthy lifestyle: www.tsirona.com/blog
- A page of free resources like e-books, guides, recipes, and challenges that I update and refresh regularly: www.tsirona.com/freestuff
- My Instagram where I post daily with bite-sized tips for living a healthy lifestyle with ease: https://www.instagram.com/tsironahealth/
- My Facebook where I post daily with tips, articles, and thoughts on living a healthy lifestyle: https://www.facebook.com/tsironahealthcoaching
- My Pinterest where I curate the best content out there to help you live your healthiest life: https://www.pinterest.com/tsirona/

OTHER BOOKS BY KELLY

You, but Better Companion Journal and Workbook

This book is a journal and workbook companion to the best-selling book, You, but Better: Stop Making Your Health So Hard! **You can use it on its own or with You, but Better.**

Struggling to maintain a healthy lifestyle while tackling life's demands? Dig deeper into your unique and personal needs for making wellness a number-one priority, even with a busy schedule.

Are you a successful woman conquering the world, but losing control of your health? Have you tried to get healthier in the past, but time constraints made it feel impossible? Have you stopped taking care of yourself to meet the responsibilities of career and family? Certified health coach, personal trainer, and fitness nutrition specialist, Dr. Kelly Morgan has helped hundreds of women set goals and reach health success while dealing with their hectic lives. Now she's here to share how to reclaim your vitality – even with your crazy busy life – to be the best, healthier person you can be.

This journal and workbook follows Dr. Morgan's proven program, You, but Better. It will help you gain the insight to develop a sustainable and manageable healthy lifestyle strategy to fit your individual needs. By following journal prompts and exercises that help you expand on Dr. Morgan's deeply researched and sensible approach, you'll gain a unique understanding of how to overcome obstacles and change defeating mindsets to create the happy, vibrant future you deserve.

In the You, but Better Journal and Workbook, you'll delve deeper into your unique needs and plan for feeling the best you ever have.

Prompts and exercises in the book span Dr. Morgan's 7 pillars of a healthy lifestyle:

- Pillar 1: Self-Examination - Honor the real star of this story—you—to get a better idea of what you want to achieve in your plan and, most importantly, why.
- Pillar 2: Goal Setting - These exercises will be the difference between what habits haven't stuck in the past and getting to the new you.
- Pillar 3: Mindset - Get your mind in the right place by focusing on useful outlooks that meld your high-achieving superpowers into tools for a healthy lifestyle that fits you.
- Pillar 4: Movement - Figure out a manageable activity routine that gets you moving more while fitting into your unique lifestyle, no matter your preferences, needs, or barriers.
- Pillar 5: Nutrition - Figure out your nutritional desires and come up with a healthy, doable plan to follow - that's still food-positive.
- Pillar 6: Stress Management - Understand what causes your stress and use that knowledge to help you manage it.
- Pillar 7: Energy Management - Work through your energy cycle and limitations. Your energy is finite, so you'll also work on not forcing yourself to "do it all," no matter how much of the world is on your shoulders.
- Now What? - Have a plan for what happens after you have reached and exceeded your goals and are beginning to set new ones.

Buy the You, but Better Journal and Workbook to restore your spark today!

Mentally Hungry: A Guided Emotional Eating Escape Plan

Do you turn to sugary junk in times of stress? Learn how to satiate your true inner desires and trade the potato chips for fabulous progress.

Has a healthy diet taken a backseat to your other priorities? Are you tired of feeling sluggish after rewarding yourself with a tasty treat? Have decadent nibbles become a dangerous crutch? Certified health coach, personal trainer, and fitness nutrition specialist, Dr. Kelly Morgan is all too familiar with the soothing nature of emotional eating during turmoil. Now she's here to show you how to steer cravings away from snacks and toward simple ways of soothing your emotions - without food.

Mentally Hungry: A Guided Emotional Eating Escape Plan is a judgment-free guide that helps busy women identify the causes of emotional eating and develop smart, productive substitutes. By looking inside and identifying personal triggers, Dr. Morgan reveals the secrets to regaining control of eating patterns. And with a food-positive, lighthearted approach easing you into change, you'll be excited to ditch the chocolate bar and confidently secure a healthier future.

In Mentally Hungry: A Guided Emotional Eating Escape Plan, you'll:

- Gain awareness of your personal emotional eating triggers and know the proper action to handle your specific problem areas
- Be able to react to the triggers in a healthy way rather than make food decisions in the moment
- Create an "if this, then that" action plan for what to do when trigger emotions and situations come up
- Be able to experience your emotions in a healthy way and deal with them without using food
- Be able to identify cravings and satisfy them in a smart and healthy way without restriction

- Have a maintenance plan that keeps emotional eating at bay for good
- Get inspiration from real-life turnaround stories, tons of practical examples, and much, much more!

Mentally Hungry: A Guided Emotional Eating Escape Plan is the perfect resource for those wanting to find a better way to feel good. If you like conversational guidance, action-oriented solutions, and small changes that make big differences, then you'll love Dr. Kelly Morgan's motivational tool.

Buy Mentally Hungry: A Guided Emotional Eating Escape Plan to satisfy your heart today!

HOW TO WORK WITH KELLY

Scan below to visit Kelly's website

- Coaching: https://www.tsirona.com/work-with-me
- Online courses: https://tsirona.teachable.com/courses
- Recipe and guided meditation subscriptions: https://www.tsirona.com/subscriptions

AFTERWORD

Please consider reviewing or just rating this book on Amazon. It helps other readers find my work. It'll count as your good deed of the day!

Scan the QR code below.

REFERENCES

1. Bachus, T. (2015). 3 secrets to forming new healthy habits. *ACE Fitness*. Retrieved from https://www.acefitness.org/education-and-resources/professional/expert-articles/5733/3-secrets-to-forming-new-healthy-habits
2. Centers for Disease Control and Prevention. (2017). Normal weight, overweight, and obesity among adults aged 20 and over, by selected characteristics: United States, selected years 1988–1994 through 2013–2016. Retrieved from https://www.cdc.gov/nchs/hus/contents2017.htm#058
3. Centers for Disease Control and Prevention. (2018). Physical activity basics. Retrieved from https://www.cdc.gov/physicalactivity/basics/index.htm?CDC_AA_refVal=https%3A%2F%2Fwww.cdc.gov%2Fcancer%2Fdcpc%2Fprevention%2Fpolicies_practices%2Fphysical_activity%2Fguidelines.htm
4. Fogg, B. J. (2012, December 5). Forget big change, start with a tiny habit [Video file]. Retrieved from https://www.youtube.com/watch?v=AdKUJxjn-R8&t=3s
5. Hasselbalch, A. L. (2010). Genetics of dietary habits and obesity - a twin study. *Danish Medical Bulletin, 57*(9), B4182.
6. Holmes, T. H., & Rahe, R. H. (1967). The social readjustment rating scale. *Journal of Psychosomatic Research, 11*, 213-218.
7. Martin, B. (2018). In-depth: Cognitive behavior therapy. *PsychCentral*. Retrieved from https://psychcentral.com/lib/in-depth-cognitive-behavioral-therapy/?all=1
8. Nakamura, J., & Csikszentmihályi, M. (2001). Flow theory and research. In C. R. Snyder, E. Wright, and S. J. Lopez (Eds.). *Handbook of Positive Psychology* (195-206). Oxford: Oxford University Press.

9. Prochaska, J. O., & Velicer, W. F. (1997). The transtheoretical model of health behavior change. *American Journal of Health Promotion, 12*(1), 38-48.
10. Reimers, C. D., Knapp, G., & Reimers, A. K. (2012). Does physical activity increase life expectancy? A review of the literature. *Journal of Aging Research, 2012*.
11. Sethi, R. (n.d.). How to master the habits of successful people. *I Will Teach You to be Rich*. https://www.iwillteachyoutoberich.com/blog/how-to-master-the-habits-of-successful-people/
12. Thaler, R. H., & Sunstein, C. R. (2008). *Nudge: Improving decisions about health, wealth, and happiness*. New Haven: Yale University Press.
13. USDA. (2018). Dietary guidelines for Americans 2015-2020. Retrieved from https://www.choosemyplate.gov/dietary-guidelines

ABOUT THE AUTHOR

Kelly Morgan, Ph.D. owns Tsirona, where she is a health coach for busy, high-achieving women who have put their health on the backburner while kicking butt in the rest of their lives. She helps women gain control of their health and use it as a tool for continuing to lead their crazy lives and achieve their big dreams. She has recovered from anorexia, gained too much weight in a time of stress, and finally discovered how to make her health much easier.

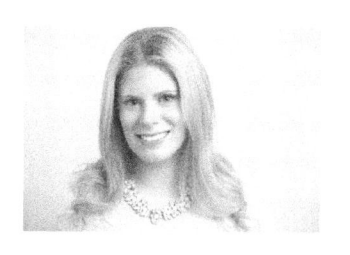

Dr. Morgan's online coaching and courses help her clients set their goals and reach success. She has been featured in media outlets such as Self, Yoga Journal, Elite Daily, and HealthyWay.

Dr. Morgan has a unique mix of formal education in writing, health communication, and business that is supplemented by her experience as a certified personal trainer, health coach, fitness nutrition specialist, and RYT 200 yoga teacher. She is also an adjunct professor in the Health and Sport Management departments at the largest university in Virginia, where she has had a near-100% success rate with guiding her hundreds of students through health behavior change projects to reach their goals.

Made in the USA
Las Vegas, NV
27 November 2023